LECTIN-FREE COOKBOOK:

30 Simple, Quick, and Easy Recipes to Help You Improve Your Health, Reduce Inflammation, Prevent Risk of a Disease, and Shield Your Gut from Lectin Damage

Table of Contents

Introduction
Chapter 1: Welcome to Lectin-Free Cooking!......1
Chapter 2: Lectin-Free Breakfast Recipes.........44

    Hashed Sweet Potatoes
    Mushroom Thyme Gravy and Lectin-Free Biscuits
    Pancakes Made With Cinnamon Cassava Flour
    Breakfast Burritos

Chapter 3: Lectin-Free Lunch Recipes..............63

    Greens and Wild Shrimp With a Zesty Lemon Oil
    Chicken Soup With Shirataki Rice
    Escarole and Shrimp Salad
    Spinach and Steak Salad
    Roasted Cobb Salad
    Meatball and Bok Choy Salad
    The Plant Patty Burger
    Lectin-Free, Vegan Taco "Meat"

Chapter 4: Lectin-Free Dinner Recipes............88

   Angel Hair Shirataki Noodles With Broiled Clams Over Them

   Avocado and Egg Over a Noodle Bowl

   Goat Cheese and Chicken Enchiladas

   The Tuna Helper Remix!

   Shepherd's Pie

   Caesar Salad (Lectin-Free Version)

   Shrimp and Broccoletti Stir-Fry Over Toasted Sesame Cauliflower Rice

   Apricot Balsamic Chicken

   Chicken Mushroom Limes

   Sirloin Steak Leeks

   Dijon Salmon Cakes

Chapter 5: Lectin-Free Dessert Recipes...........131

   Summer-Time Strawberry Short Cake

   Lectin-Free Blueberry Fools

Chapter 6: Lectin-Free Snack Recipes............138

   Coconut Wrapped Raviolis

   Fresh Rainbow Fries (From the Oven)

Great Mashed Potatoes Alternatives!
Pickled Celery From the Fridge
Multi-Seed Grain-Free Bread

Conclusion……………………………………………..156
Description

© Copyright 2018 by Layla Grant - All rights reserved.

The following eBook is reproduced below with the goal of providing information that is as accurate and reliable as possible. Regardless, purchasing this eBook can be seen as consent to the fact that both the publisher and the author of this book are in no way experts on the topics discussed within and that any recommendations or suggestions that are made herein are for entertainment purposes only. Professionals should be consulted as needed prior to undertaking any of the action endorsed herein.

This declaration is deemed fair and valid by both the American Bar Association and the Committee of Publishers Association and is legally binding throughout the United States.

Furthermore, the transmission, duplication, or reproduction of any of the following work including specific information will be considered an illegal act irrespective of if it is done electronically or in print. This extends to creating a secondary or tertiary copy of the work or a recorded copy and is only allowed with express written consent from the Publisher. All additional right reserved.

The information in the following pages is broadly considered to be a truthful and accurate account of facts, and as such any inattention, use, or misuse of the information in question by the reader will render any resulting actions solely under their purview. There are no scenarios in which the publisher or the original author of this work can be in any fashion deemed liable for any hardship or damages that may befall them after undertaking information described herein.

Additionally, the information in the following pages is intended only for informational purposes and should thus be thought of as universal. As befitting its nature, it is presented without assurance regarding its prolonged validity or interim quality. Trademarks that are mentioned are done without written consent and can in no way be considered an endorsement from the trademark holder.

Introduction

Congratulations on downloading *LECTIN-FREE COOKBOOK: 30 Simple, Quick, and Easy Recipes to Help You Improve Your Health, Reduce Inflammation, Prevent Risk of a Disease, and Shield Your Gut from Lectin Damage* and thank you for doing so.

The following chapters will help you start a lectin-free diet that'll help you become a better version of you! We will be going over 30 different yummy recipes that will help you live the healthier life that you've been wanting. For those of you who are new to the lectin-free diet, we'll also briefly be going over the science and reasoning behind the diet.

From it's beginning with Dr. Gundry's research, lectin-free eating has quickly become one of the most sought out diets of our time. Even singing sensation Kelly Clarkson has vouched for the diet! As someone who's publicly struggled with their weight, Clarkson understands the struggles of trying to start a healthier lifestyle. We'll explore her story and many others in this book. Hopefully, reading their stories will give you the drive you need to start living a better life with lectin-free dieting today.

Join millions of people see and feel the changes in your body. With this new diet, you'll be sleeping better than you have in years. You'll feel your waist getting a little trimmer. You'll notice that you have more energy than before. Who knows! Maybe, you'll be able to give up caffeine. That is if you happen to love it like more of the world seems to!

Our recipes will make it easier for you to keep in line with the diet as well. These recipes were picked not just because they tend to be lectin-free recipes, but because they're great alternatives to some of the tastiest meals you've had growing up.

So, sit back, enjoy the photos, the foods, and the information because we're going to change the way you look at cooking and dieting forever!

There are plenty of books on this subject on the market, thanks again for choosing this one! Every effort was made to ensure it is full of as much useful information as possible, please enjoy!

Amazon review would be always appreciate it so much ☺

Chapter 1: Welcome to Lectin-Free Cooking!

Diet trends come and go, but lectin-free dieting is proving to be more than a mere fad! Unlike other diets, where there's a super extensive list of what you can and cannot eat, to the point where it feels like it's setting you up for familiar, lectin-free dieting isn't like that.

In his book, *The Plant Paradox*, M.D. Steven Gundry, who's a cardiologist and heart surgeon who works in Southern California, has built a dietary empire with one simple claim. He claims that any food with the plant protein lectin should be avoided. It's your worst enemy or your body's worst enemy. It especially hinders your ability to lose weight.

It is a slippery slope as lectins are found in many things that we consume on a daily basis. They're in stuff like our whole grains, squashes, tomatoes, beans, nuts, and many of the animal proteins that we consume. There are quite a few more, but that'll give you an idea of what we mean.

Gundry makes the claim that we humans aren't meant to eat foods that contain lectins. If we happen to eliminate their intake, then we can reduce stuff like inflammation of the body, lose weight, and overall lead ourselves to a healthier lifestyle.

So, what are lectins?

The scientific definition of lectins, according to PrecisionNutrition.com, is *"thought to play a role in immune function, cell growth, cell death, and body fat regulation. Because we don't digest lectins, we often produce antibodies to them. Almost everyone has antibodies to some dietary lectins in their body. This means our responses vary. Certain foods can even become intolerable to someone after an immune system change, or the gut is injured from another source. The presence of particular lectins can stimulate an immune system response. There are some lectins that no one should consume. Ever wonder why you don't see sprouted red kidney beans?*

It's due to phytohaemagglutinin – a lectin that can cause red kidney bean poisoning. The poisoning is usually caused by the ingestion of raw, soaked kidney beans. As few as four or five raw beans can trigger symptoms.
Raw kidney beans contain from 20,000 to 70,000 lectin units, while fully cooked beans usually contain between 200 and 400 units."

With all the science talk, they sound like they're positive for the body. And while science is still figuring out the yes and no of the complicated situation, Dr. Gundry has proven that excessive amounts of the stuff can be the reason why we suffer from certain problems.

Lectins are proteins that you'll naturally find in many foods you see at the store. Grains and beans have lectin in them. They tend to bind together your carbohydrates. Ideally, they can help your cells interact and communicate with one another. In the plants we eat, Dr. Gundry said in an interview that they're plants that protect themselves against being eaten. He said that by making insects and animals feel sick to their stomach, these lectins make it so that the pest doesn't want to eat anything that is lectin-filled ever again.

Gundry said in the interview: "Anytime a diet starts to take out a massive amount of food groups, it's a little faddish by nature."

Gundry notes that eating lectins provokes an inflammatory response within the body. This sadly can lead to weight gain and some other serious health conditions like that of a leaky gut or irritable bowel syndrome.

And what exactly is this so-called lectin-free diet?

According to a dietitian named Amy Goodson: "The lectin-free diet takes out high-lectin foods like grains, quinoa, legumes, and nightshade vegetables like tomatoes, peppers, and eggplant." This also means that you'll want to avoid things such as dairy, fruit that's out of season, and meat and chicken that hasn't been pastured or grass-fed prior to their slaughter. You'll want to avoid conventionally raised animals basically.

You'll want to add new things to your diet. Gundry's diet suggests that you get a plate with low-lectin based food such as leafy green vegetables such as cauliflower, broccoli, asparagus, mushroom, seeds and nuts, millet, meats that have been pasture-raised, and wildly caught fish and shrimp and such.

As a personal testament to the diet's work, Gundry says that he lost 70 pounds on his lectin-free diet. His patients that he's put on the diet can also attest to this.

"The amazing thing is when people change nothing except removing major lectins, they start losing weight, and they still are eating lots of calories, but we're not storing it as fat anymore," Gundry said in the interview.

There's a 2006 study that Dr. Gundry leans on for his lectin-free diet. The results indicated that there was a positive effect on people when they stopped eating lectin. People who had cardiovascular disease and metabolic syndrome evidently felt better. These are people who suffer from having increased blood pressure, high blood sugar levels, extra body fat located normally around the waist, and abnormally high or low cholesterol levels.

Dr. Gundry's lectin-free diet hasn't been without its naysayers, with one professional, Samantha Cassetty, R.D., saying that lectins can be really beneficial to weight loss. She cited a 2017 study that mentioned that whole grains were associated with weight loss. Yet another study was published saying that people who had eaten pulses over a 6-week period, meaning they consumed beans, lentils, and chickpeas, for example, had lost a surprising amount of weight in comparison to those who didn't eat any pulses.

But the proof is there. Another professional, Leah Kaufman, R.D., who have specified that she's seen weight loss success in some patients who suffer from irritable bowel syndrome after they went on a low-lectin diet. Lectins are even reportedly problematic in higher quantities as well, especially if you eat the food raw.

Regardless of the back and forth between scientists on rather we should or should not be eating lectin-based foods, one very popular persona has come forth and given her stamp of approval: Kelly Clarkson!

Known for winning the first-ever American Idol contest back in the early 2000s, Kelly Clarkson has made a name for herself in the music career. With a 15-year career that continues to show her a successful female artist, Ms. Clarkson has had her shares of up and downs. She's been pretty vocal, pun intended, about her troubled relationship with her father, but one of the most public things she'd had to deal with is struggling with her weight.

Clarkson has constantly been then a success story and the butt-end of awful fat jokes over her career.

"Even on American Idol I was really thin, but I was bigger than the other girls on the show, so people would say things to me," she told People magazine in an interview in 2018. "But luckily I am super confident, so I've never had a problem with shutting people down and saying, 'Yeah, you know, that's just what I'm rocking. It's fine.'"

She's currently losing weight, and it's with the help of Dr. Gundry's diet.

In a blog post on his site, in mid-June, he wrote: "Did you happen to hear about the Kelly Clarkson diet on The Today Show? She looked amazing. Not that she isn't always beautiful, she is. But recently, the singer lost 37 pounds by following a cutting-edge diet called The Plant Paradox. That's not an easy feat for a mother of four who works full time. [...] How did it happen? Well, Ms. Clarkson said she read the book The Plant Paradox. [...] 'It's basically about how we cook our food, non-GMO, no pesticides, eating really organic,' said the singer. After applying the principles of the diet to her own lifestyle, Clarkson was even able to turn her health around. Everybody's talking about the amazing Kelly Clarkson weight loss plan. But, it's not just about losing weight."

If Kelly Clarkson's testimonial wasn't enough for you, then perhaps you'd like to hear more from other people who've said that lectin-free eating has changed their lives.

One lady, by the name of Michelle, discussed her eating allergies and tells how lectin-free eating changed her life.

She writes that she had found out that she had Celiac's disease. She also suffers from thyroid disease and rheumatoid arthritis. She claims that she's allergic to dairy products and they have spent a portion of her life avoiding all of that alongside peanut butter, sesame seeds, cranberries, and lamb and beef. Things got complicated once she found how that she had to be gluten-free now. She had to void rye, barley, wheat, and sometimes oats. She was surprised to have realized that most grains actually have gluten in them, especially corn, she exclaims. She says that she's going to switch to a grain-free diet and helps that her system will be able to improve so that she can no longer rely on her medication.

As far lectins go, she had started researching the diet and was wondering what all the commotion was about. She advises people to remove all highly toxic foods that have lectin in them for their diet as soon as possible. She then hopes that people will slowly add one food group in at a time. It'll help them to see which one new dieters are sensitive to if not all. She herself has to avoid nightshade vegetables because they were advised against her R.A. She strongly advises people to get rid of corn from their diet. Her advice for dieters is pretty sound.

"Remove beans/legumes (including soy and peanuts) and also remove all dairy. Lactose-free milk still contains dairy, so I would switch to almond because it is the safest and it's super delicious. Especially the Diamond Valley brand in the refrigerator section."

She tells readers that after they've eliminated all of these things for about 10 days, they can introduce the least toxic ones back into their diets. That way, they'll see that affects them in which way. The bottom line is, she writes, that is you have a bad reaction to it, then don't eat it. Eventually, introduce dairy and then eventually legumes and beans into your body and finally grains.

What her testimony tells us is that lectin-free dieting isn't just dieting, it's a way to cook healthier for yourself. Perhaps, you're like her, and you're allergic to certain foods like peanuts. Perhaps, you have to live a gluten-free life as well. Either way, our recipes take into consideration a wide variety of people. Some people will continue to eat meat, and others want to avoid anything associated with animals. That's fine! Let us help!

Other people responded to the forum, giving their support and insight into her story.

Another forum writer says that they were really interested in the lectin story and felt a sense of kinship to it. They realized that lectin was a concern for them as well. They were taking a protein-digesting aid that acted as an enzyme that helped to deconstruct their food. Additionally, they also took a prebiotic mix with L-glutamine, which are known for helping to repair one's gut lining and help aid in obtaining a better immune system. They also are note taking a probiotic and a supplement that is called "lectin control." It helps the body in maintaining lectins.

The writer avoids dairy in most cases and also avoids gluten, nightshades, and even soy. They have to avoid certain fruits as well, such as pears, apples, grapes, and kiwi. They also have to avoid beans, though they do say that they're okay with consuming lentils as long as it's not part of their everyday diet. When they accidentally slip up here and there, they notice that their body has some bloating.

In the end, the writer concludes that: "*It's really elimination and then tries reintroducing them if you react then wait at least 6-12 months before trying to reintroduce again. Also, I am a huge believer in positive thinking, if you started to get down and stressed about what you can't eat, you end up becoming more intolerant to other things, whereas if you focus on the foods, you can eat and keep positive. Hopefully you will be able to tolerate them again.
I must admit I find breaky really hard.*"

The conversation about lectin-free eating is growing, and more and more people are becoming apart of the bigger conversation started by Dr. Gundry. It's waking up many people to something in our foods that we've been unaware of for years.

Another people on the forum discuss their recent concerns with some of the products that they've seen on their local store's shelves. They're worried about the dairy lectins within the U.S. At the time of writing the post, the writer was 3 months removed from moving to the United States. They note that they're going for a difference in their meat eating as well. They note the difference between eating a grass-fed cow in comparison to eating products that come from cows from which you are not sure what they were eating prior to their slaughter. They were considering taking some packages of EasiYo with them when they leave. It would be used for making their own yogurt. It's their main source of dairy consumption. They also eat stuff like coconut milk-based ice cream and rice milk or almond milk as a substitution for regular cow's milk.

The writer makes note of giving up high-lectin contain foods. They did so in the following order: gluten grains, soy, nightshades, citrus, though they do wonder if they think that eventually, they get back to eating citrus-based foods at some point, all legumes, which they note as including green beans and fresh green peas, peanut butter, and peanuts. It wasn't completely easy for the writer to go cold turkey with them. They had to slowly get them out of their diet by eating them in limited amounts before they were able to kick them out of their diet entirely. They're concerned that there isn't enough research being done on lectins.

This forum writer brings up a good point. Lectins, we know, are being researched, but it's through Dr. Gundry's research, analysis, and diet that we're truly learning more about them. With this lectin-free diet becoming a mainstay in today's diet market, other researchers have no choice but to look at what is being said about it and make the concern for more research a bigger priority. That being said, the writer, does give their personal opinion on lectin-free dieting debate. They consider gluten in corn to be different other gluten-based grains. It is, however, high in lectins, they say. Their belief is that the problem many people are having with barley, rye, and wheat is due to the lectins in them, not the gluten per say. They find the commonality of people struggling with this as people have similar problems with dairy, corn, soy, etc.

As we see here, this writer concerns themselves with what animals are put to slaughter are few prior to getting on to our shelves. They're right, consumers do not know what they've been eating. Perhaps, their food was lectin heavy, which once digested into them gives the chance that you too will consume these lectins. We've already mentioned how science is concerned about the body having excessive lectin in it.

For some people, as you'll read in this next forum post, lectin-free dieting has become a great alternative for those who are allergic to dairy-based products.

"I cannot tolerate dairy and neither can my daughter, although its hard to stop her, I try to limit how much she has, otherwise she gets awful wind.
I do have issues with Soy, and Beans, although I am ok with peas and green beans, I am also ok with lentils.

It would be really good to hear of more research been done with lectins. I have found after 12 months of no potatoes, I can tolerate in very small moderation, I pinched a couple of my daughter's hot chips the other day and didn't end up bloated and in pain.

It is hard to limit all of them although I do believe once we have improved our digestive system and immune system and the cells in the intestinal wall have improved it is possible to tolerate some of these foods again.
Good luck with your travels, I hope you are able to keep eating the way you have been."

What's great about lectin-free diet is that it gives you many alternatives to dairy-based products. We're proud to say that we've added a few great alternatives in these recipes for you to read! In some cases, the alternative even has more nutritional value than their dairy counterparts!

What about people who are suffering from various medical conditions? What does the research say? Can Dr. Gundry's diet help? For another forum writer, the answer is yes!

"Hello all, after having sent myself crazy with the tons of research and conflicting info on the net, I decided to look for a book where I might get the info I needed, and I found it here.

I suffer from Psoriasis and Psoriatic Arthritis and seeking to follow a lectin free diet from now on and can definitely use some help and guidance.

So recently one of my friends who also suffers from Psoriasis brought up the issue of "lectins," and certain sources are showing that peas/beans need to be pressurized to get rid of the lectins, other sources are showing that all peas/beans are lectin free, so you can see my utter confusion, Anyway, guys, I can tell you once
I found this book I was completely saved! I'm no longer confused, and I have an easy to follow guide that I can just open up and prepare any meal needed."

The success stories continue on!

A different forum writer claimed herself to be a thankful, energetic, active, healthy woman. After she started her lectin-free dieting journey, she noticed that she was already feeling better than she could put into words within the first week.

From then on, she noticed that she was getting better each and every day. She went from having a body that was wracked with pain, having a digestive mess that harmed her mentally (she was suffering from memory loss and having moments where she'd space out. She recalls never being able to sleep more than an hour or so at one point and collectively only sleep for like five hours. It ran her ragged. But once she changed her diet, she was able to get back to living her life. She started working full time again, which was the first time she could do so in many years. She started to organize and clean her house, something that she's wanted to do for years now as well. She never had enough energy to keep up with her kids, and that made it difficult for her. She now exercises daily, as she rides her bike for about 10 to 20 miles a day now! At the time of writing her post, she was planning on going skiing yet again!

Her testimonial paints a great picture of what can be in store for you when you embrace the lectin-free cooking diet. She mentions that she was able to run a marathon within her first month of doing the diet. She left many of her loved ones speechless. They were used to seeing a woman who had spent most of her life sick. In retrospect, she sees that she was even sicker than she initially thought. She recently, at the time of writing that is, celebrated the victory of a positive blood test results reading. She was not only doing better with her vitamin intake but was actually excelling at eating healthier. All because she started and has stayed on the lectin-free diet.

"For years I had mouth sores, terrible gas, some diarrhea, occasional anemia, DH and various other symptoms. Then, during a bout of terrible anemia, I went downhill horribly. Liver functions out of whack, daily fevers up to 105 (that went on for weeks), everything I ate tasted like metal, inability to think or carry on a

conversation, alternating chills and hot flashes, eventually unable to walk by myself. All of which led to hospitalization for 11 days and completely missing 10 weeks of work. Doctors were sure I had non-Hodgkins lymphoma. Another thought my liver was failing. It was undiagnosed celiac.

It was months before I was "normal" and back to strength again, but every single one of those problems was solved by going lectin-free."

"My hubby and I are doing our best to eliminate all lectins after reading your (or someone else's?) original post about lectins and after doing some online research. I was already soy free and nightshade free, and seem to have naturally gravitated (since going gluten-free) to foods that do not contain lectins anyway, so it is not that difficult. Just meant avoiding all canola oil, cutting out peanut butter (a biggy for hubby) and reinforcing what had become a

natural avoidance of legumes. I kept thinking I should be eating more legumes and kept finding reasons not to use them somehow :o , and now I think my subconscious was telling me I did not respond well to them. And here white bean salad used to be one of my favorite salads. Haven't made it in ages. And split pea soup was a favorite since it was most often gluten-free.

Hubby has been fighting sinus congestion for a long time, even after he completed his series of shots for grass allergies, and since eliminating the lectins, he says they are quite clear now. I had been once again having nighttime bloating and racing heart, and since cutting out lectins, going back on digestive enzymes and taking a Motilium at bedtime it has so far not recurred. Of course, we don't know which (or if it's the combination) is helping, but these episodes were so distressing I am not willing to experiment.

I was surprised that I had never really heard of lectins before, but then I hadn't heard much about gluten either."

"Okay so after going gluten-free I had an improvement in some symptoms, and then others got worse. So, after a little online research, I decided to go lectin free as well. I'm in my first week of that and feel a huge difference although the diet feels very restrictive. I'm going to start challenging things soon and hopefully will add a few things back in.
Anyway... are there any others here who are lectin free as well? I read that lectin is similar to gluten so a lot of people who react to gluten (which is a lectin group) will react to the other lectin families as well like the nightshades, dairy or legumes."

One testimonial mentioned by another forum writer said that they were on the lectin-free diet for long enough that they were able to see great results happening to their body. They're on the lucky ones, they say, who didn't have to wait years, misdiagnoses, and other such things to get where they are. They had acute symptoms happen pretty instantly after they had a terrible combination of the flu and strep throat thing happening. Their doctor told them that that was the theory behind many of the autoimmune issues and that they were "jump started" by another systemic infection.

Their situation was literally painful. They spent about three or four months dealing with bad cramps, diarrhea, headaches, and other problems. The writer says that they took a blood test and their doctor suggested that they go on a lectin-free diet. They did want their doctor said, and within a week, they felt like they were a new person! One of the things they noticed was that within a few weeks, their hip pain was gone—not just numbed but completely gone. This was one of the pains that they had each night they went to sleep. They also mentioned that their headaches were gone now too. Perhaps, the most surprising thing revealed in this testimony is that the blurriness in their eyes that they had dealt with went away and, therefore, they no longer needed their prescription glasses! The writer concludes that they are now living a cramp-free, pain-free life. They admit to having times in which they feel weak and want to cheat, but they remind themselves of what life was like when they weren't on the lectin-free diet. It was a life of pain. They never want to go back to living that way ever again.

"I went lectin free, and I have been lectin free for 2 weeks now. My first three days were amazing! I never slept so well in my entire life! I lead a

very busy social life, and I've felt silly having to ask people what they are cooking so that I can take my own food along if necessary. But I must do what will make me feel better in the end, and most of my friends have picked up this book so they already know what I can and can't eat.

But besides all that, I've lost some weight, I feel lighter than I've ever felt, my IBS is almost non-existent, and I have more energy on little sleep while being lectin free than I ever did before.

I hope you have people around you to support you and encourage you! That will help a lot. My wonderful husband will often eat the same as me when I have to pack in my own food to eat at socials events. He reminds me often that its a process to get better, but that it's completely worth it!"

A different forum writer said in their story that they have had a history of problematic issues in their life. They had Fibromyalgia, Irritable Bowel Syndrome, diabetes, low blood sugar, and even digestive issues. Talk about a laundry list of issues! At the time of posting, the writer got deathly ill during that previous fall and summer, and their doctors began to think that of these previous diagnoses weren't correct. They did some more digging into the research, and the writer was diagnosed as having Celiac Disease in late 2010. Since that then, they've been lectin-free, and they wrote that all of the problems that they had previously had gone away!

In looking further into their diagnosis, the writer reveals that they apparently had a smaller form of the disease their whole life. It fluctuated and had been a problem for them since they were six years of age! That's around the time that their hypoglycemia started. Now, it's much more manageable with their diet change.

Being lectin-free, for this individual, is really only problematic when they are in public because many restaurants, friends, and family aren't aware of the issues with lectin and therefore tend to cook foods that are high in lectin. The good news is that they're communicating with friends and family, so they're slowly learning how to adapt their cooking habits to help aid the writer in their healthier lifestyle. Most of the time, they tend to just take their own food to the places. They've found the growing amount of lectin-free recipe to be diversely helpful in bringing their own dishes to get-togethers. And yet again, that's where these 30 recipes will come in handy for you. It's not just about making them for yourself. It's about making them so that you can share them with others and inspire them too to change the way they eat.

"My first three days were amazing! I never slept so well in my entire life! I lead a very busy social life, and I've felt silly having to ask people

what they are cooking so that I can take my own food along if necessary. But I must do what will make me feel better in the end, and most of my friends have picked up this book so they already know what I can and can't eat.

But besides all that, I've lost some weight, I feel lighter than I've ever felt, my IBS is almost non-existent, and I have more energy on little sleep while being lectin free than I ever did before.

I hope you have people around you to support you and encourage you! That will help a lot. My wonderful husband will often eat the same as me when I have to pack in my own food to eat at socials events. He reminds me often that its a process to get better, but that it's completely worth it!"

This is what awaits you in the world of lectin-free dieting. You can be like one of these people and learn how to live without inflammation and other problems that come up from lectin-free dieting.

*Special note: While we are excited for you to start your lectin-free dieting, we do want to let you know that this book nor the diet itself should be considered a replacement for treatments for your medical problems. Changing one's diet can definitely help, but you should always, always make sure to consult your doctor before making any changes to your diet or lifestyle.

We recommend and even with reading this that you'll be open to doing your own research on the lectin-free diet as well. The Internet is a great place where you'll find many other forum responses and research based on the lectin diet. You may want to start your research with the man himself, Dr. Gundry. His website, *gundrymd.com*, has become (for some people) the holy grail of lectin-free diet information. Not only does the site keep the reader informed regarding the ongoing news and research about lectin-free dieting but you'll also get more tips and recipes as more and more people are becoming inventive with the diet each day. You can even read up more on Kelly Clarkson's diet and how she's quickly become the "it" girl of lectin-free dieting.

There is also a lot of research coming out of the other places that will help you make a conscious decision on what to do.

Chapter 2: Lectin-Free Breakfast Recipes

Hashed Sweet Potatoes

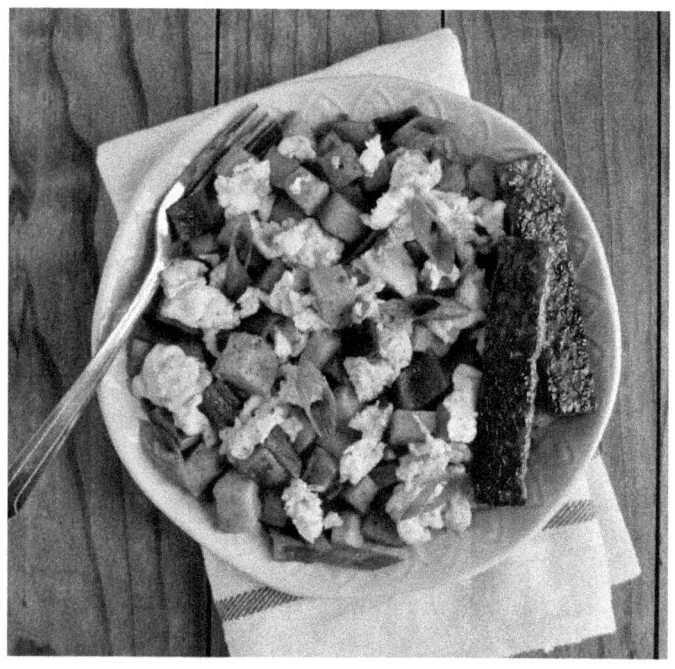

Is there a better way to start the day off than a hearty breakfast? As much as we'd love to have that good old greasy, lectin-heavy breakfast of our childhoods, it's just simply not healthy. Luckily, there are breakfast alternatives like this. They're made to fill you up and leave you feeling satiated without the unwanted inflammation and such.

This recipe makes roughly 2-4 servings and has a total time of preparation and cooking of 50 minutes.

Here's what's inside of it:
- Sliced scallions (the green part of it only)
- Minced garlic (2 cloves)
- Ground black pepper (0.25-0.50 tsp)
- Onion powder (0.5 tsp)
- Sea salt (0.5 tsp)
- Turmeric (0.5 tsp)
- Smoked paprika (1 tsp)
- Your choice of either avocado oil or olive oil (2 tbsp)

- Medium-sized sweet potatoes that have been cubed and peeled into smaller pieces (2)

Here's how you make it:
- Turn on your oven to 400 degrees Fahrenheit.
- Depending on personal preference, choose a large or medium-sized bowl, place your cubed pieces of sweet potato and oil into it, and toss about until cubes are well coated.
- Add your turmeric, paprika, onion, powder, black pepper, and sea salt between 2 pans. This will help prevent the potatoes from steaming.
- Bake the contents for about 20 minutes.
- Take the pan off the oven and place the sweet potatoes. The contents are very soft, so make sure to be gentle when handling it. (If not, you'll end up with mashed potatoes!)

- Return the pan back to your oven for between 10 and 15 minutes.
- Take the pan off the oven again and put in your minced garlic. You're in your last 5 minutes of cooking! Warning: Be sure to turn off the oven if your potatoes begin to get too dark. You can also prop your oven open to let some of the heat out.
- Don't overcook the garlic. If you can smell its presence in the contents, then it's done!
- Take contents out of the oven and place your green scallions on top.
- If you'd like to make it a fuller breakfast, then add a tofu scramble or some scrambled eggs and even some tempeh bacon!

Mushroom Thyme Gravy and Lectin-Free Biscuits

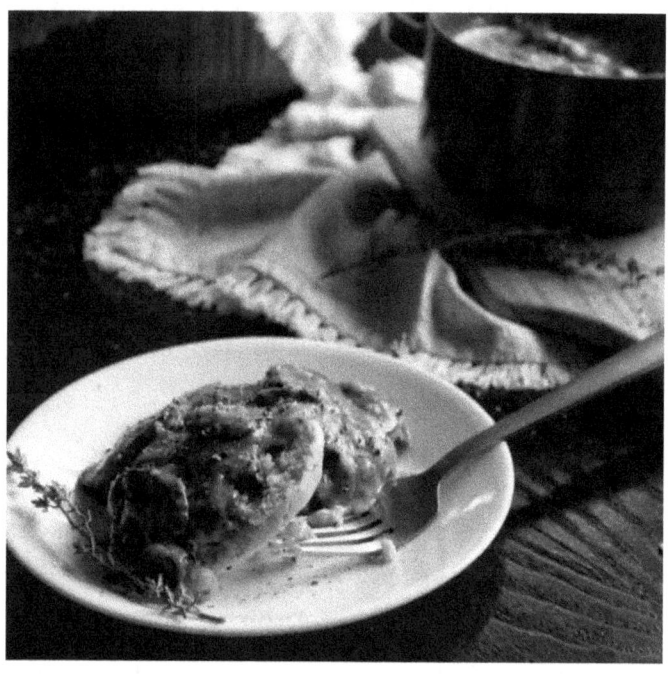

Who says you can't have your morning style biscuits and gravy anymore? Anyone from the south will tell you how essential this dish is to those lazy summer days as the cicadas sing their songs and the humid heat continues to breathe its way into the atmosphere. This time, however, we're keeping it lectin-free.

This recipe makes eight biscuits which are about 3-4 servings and has a total preparation time of one hour.

Here's what's inside the lectin-free biscuits:
- Apple cider vinegar (1 tsp)
- Light coconut milk (1.5 cups)
- Coconut oil (0.25 cup)
- Baking soda (0.5 tsp)
- Salt (1 tsp)
- Nutrient-rich yeast (2 tbsp)
- Baking powder (4 tsp)
- Sorghum flour (0.25 cup)
- Cassava flour (1.75 cups)

Here's what's inside the Mushroom Thyme Nutmeg Gravy:
- Salt (To your liking)

- Ground nutmeg (0.13-0.25 tsp)
- Sage that's been rubbed and dried (0.5 tsp)
- Cracked black pepper (0.75 and preferably fresh)
- Thyme (1 tsp either dried or fresh)
- Arrowroot starch (1.5 tbsp)
- Divided olive oil (2 tbsp)
- Full-fat coconut milk (0.5 cup)
- Mushroom broth (1.5 cups)
- Minced garlic (3 cloves, 2 tbsp)
- Your choice of a yellow or sweet onion (0.5 and diced)
- Cremini mushrooms (1 lb., sliced)

How to make the lectin-free biscuits:

- Get a small bowl and put your coconut oil in it. Then put it into the refrigerator for around 15 or so minutes. The oil should be firmed up.
- Grease your cookie sheet lightly with a thin layer of coconut oil.

- Preheat your oven to 400 degrees Fahrenheit.
- Grab a mason jar or a blender and shake up or blend your coconut milk and apple cider vinegar together. Set it aside.
- Grab a large mixing bowl and add the contents of salt, baking soda, yeast, baking powder, sorghum flour, and cassava flour together. Whisk until contents are well mixed.
- Cut off a solidly chilled piece of butter off into your dry ingredients slowly, with one chunk at a time. Use your hands to mix both of them together, taking the bigger chunks, breaking them down, and then mashing both parts together, but not completely together. If done correctly, there will be larger sized flakes left behind.
- Create a crevice in the center of the concoction and pour in a majority of the

coconut buttermilk, but not all of it! Leave roughly a few tablespoons in the cup.

- Stir the contents together until all parts are well mixed and wet. Only add the rest of the liquid if the dough is crumbly. The dough should stick together but still dry enough to handle with your hands.
- Use a 0.3-cup measuring cup to grab scoops of dough out of your bigger chunk of dough. Take the small piece into your hand and round it out. Put the uncooked biscuit onto your already-greased cookie sheet and lightly flatten it to about 1.5-inch thickness. Continue this process until you've used up all the dough.
- To help them rise, have the biscuits lightly touch one another as they cook and rise.
- Put the cookie sheet into your oven and bake the biscuits at 400 degrees Fahrenheit for around 15-20 minutes. Be sure to check them around the 15-minute mark. If the centers are still wet, put that back into the oven for close to 5 minutes.

The edges of your biscuit should be light golden brown, and the centers should be soft. Make sure the centers aren't mushy.
- Let your biscuits sit and cool themselves down for a minimum of 5 minutes. Enjoy!

How to make the gravy:
- Grab a large and deep pot, the ones usually used for soups, over a medium level heat. Let heat up a bit and then add 1 tablespoon of olive oil, then your onions, and then a sprinkle of salt. Stirring the contents occasionally, let the onions begin to brown and become sort of translucent. Taste for overall preference of saltiness and add a little more in desired.
- Add your minced garlic and let the contents cook for about another 2 minutes. Garlic should be slightly golden.
- Take your contents and put into your choice blender or processor and pour in the mushroom broth, coconut milk, a sprinkle of salt, black pepper, and

arrowroot starch. Blend all of this together until contents are a rich liquid and then put it aside.

- Grab your pan from earlier and put it on the stove again over a high-level heat. Add 1 tablespoon of coconut oil or your olive oil. Then add another sprinkle of salt, nutmeg, sage, and mushrooms together.

- Your mushrooms should be cooked until the moisture they excrete has evaporated. This will take probably about 10 minutes. Once evaporated, lower the heat to medium to prevent them from over-cooking. Stir a few times until your mushrooms are noticeably smaller and lightly golden-brown. This should happen within 7 or so minutes.

- Add your broth to the pot once your mushrooms are done. Return the heat back to high and make sure you're constantly stirring it! Your mixture will begin to lightly boil and will thicken a bit when it's done.

- Take the time to test taste your contents. Add more salt if you think it lacks saltiness. Add more thyme and sage if you think it needs a bit of an herbal kick. Add nutmeg if you want to be festive!

When both are done:
- Cut your biscuits in half and put as much of the gravy you desire onto each side. Be sure to store the remaining gravy into a sealed container and place in the fridge. Contents should last for about 3 days. Biscuits should be put in a Ziploc bag and stored on a counter in your kitchen. These also could last for about three days.
- Special note on mushrooms: Certain mushrooms will cook faster or slower than others, so make sure to keep a good eye on them as you're cooking them!

Pancakes Made with Cinnamon Cassava Flour

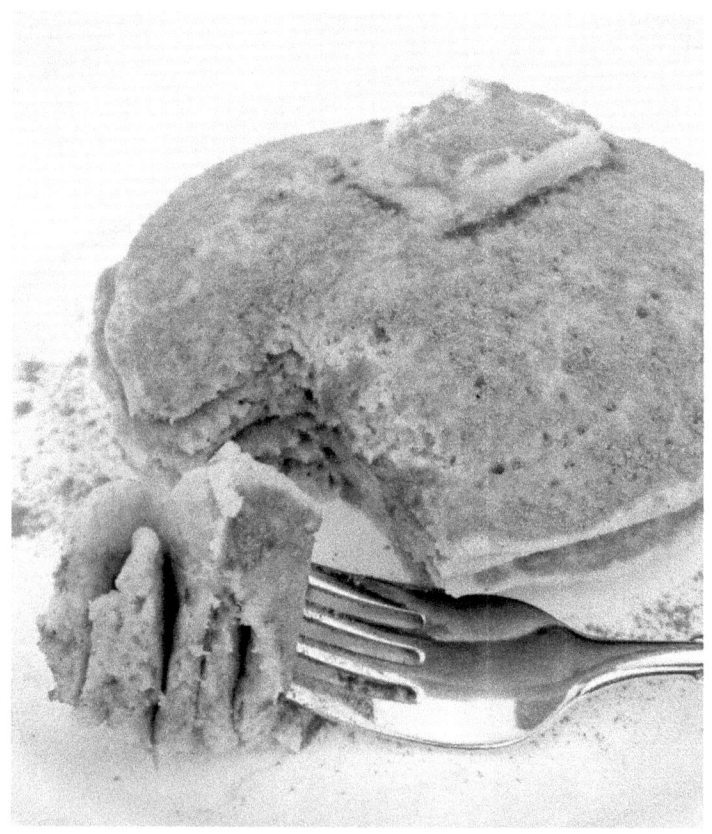

Did you really think that you were going to have to get rid of your pancakes? No way! Here's how you can still have you breakfast traditions, but it's given a lectin-free spin!

This recipe has a total of 35 minutes including the preparation and cooking time. It serves about four people.

Here's what's inside the recipe:
- Water (0.25 cup)
- Melted butter (3 tbsp and more that'll be used for serving)
- Large eggs at room temperature (2)
- Vanilla extract (0.5 tsp)
- Almond or Coconut yogurt at room temperature (1.25 cups)
- Nutmeg (0.13 tsp)
- Sea salt (0.25 tsp)
- Cinnamon (1 tsp and more for when you're serving)
- Baking powder (1 tbsp)

- Monk's fruit sweetener (2 tbsp)
- Cassava flour (1 cup)

Here's how you'll make them:
- Get your griddle and preheat to medium-low heat.
- Get your flour, sweetener, baking powder, cinnamon, sea salt, and nutmeg and whisk them together in a medium bowl until combined.
- Then whisk together your kefir/yogurt, vanilla, eggs, and water in a large bowl until all contents are combined.
- Whisk butter into your kefir mixture.
- COMBINE your dry contents with the wet mixture into a large bowl. Whisk the contents until it is smooth and combined.
- Grab a 0.25 measuring cup to pour your batter onto the heated griddle.
- Make roughly 1-3 pancakes at a time.

- Cook the pancakes until smaller bubbles break the top and on the sides.
- Pancakes are ready when there's a golden-brown tone to them, which will take about 2 minutes.
- Flip them with your spatula and cook them for about 1 minute more.
- Repeat this process with the rest of your batter.
- SERVE them hot or cover them with a clean, moist kitchen cloth to keep them from drying out.

Sprinkle some cinnamon on top and serve them with butter.

Breakfast Burritos

Many breakfasts around the world are wrapped up and ready to go within a short amount of time. Luckily, with the lectin-free diet, you can still rush out the door with a breakfast burrito like nothing in your life has changed, except that you're on the road to a healthier lifestyle.

The total time it'll take to prepare, and cook is about 15 minutes. It makes four servings.

Here's what you'll need for the recipe:
- 6-8 inched cassava flour tortillas (8 of them)
- Crumbled goat's cheese (4 oz)
- Eggs that have been beaten (6)
- Himalayan sea salt and black pepper
- Thinly sliced garlic (2 cloves)
- Chopped spinach (2 oz)

- Extra-virgin olive oil (2 tbsp)

Here's how you'll make it:
- Heat your oil into a large skillet over the medium heat.
- Add your 0.25 pepper, 0.50 tsp of salt, garlic, and spinach and cook them until the spinach wilts. It'll take about 2-3 minutes. Spread them evenly across your pan.
- Get your eggs and pour them over the spinach and garlic. Let it rest for 30 seconds. Then chop and scramble the eggs about the pan with a spatula for about 3-4 minutes.
- Turn off the heat and spread some goat cheese onto the eggs and let it soften.
- In the meantime, heat your tortillas in the microwave, making sure that they're covered by the damp towel to keep them from drying out. Heat four of them at a time, 30 seconds each time.

- Grab a spoon and put the eggs at the center of each tortilla, fold them over, and enjoy!

Chapter 3: Lectin-Free Lunch Recipes

Greens and Wild Shrimp with a Zesty Lemon Oil

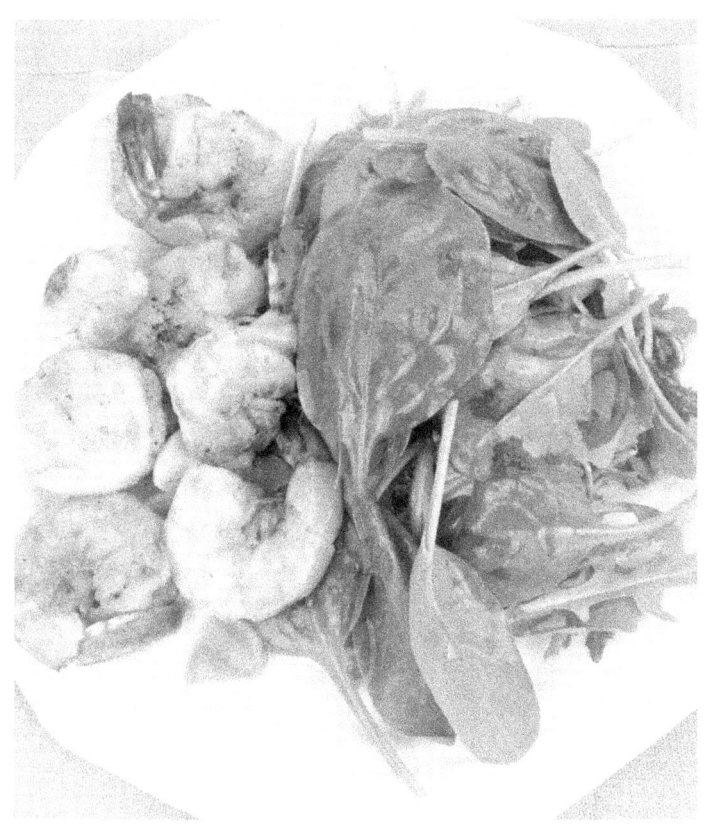

If you love shrimp, you're going to love this dish! You won't even think that you're on a diet because of how savory and zesty this dish. You can even trick your friends into eating a lectin-free diet! Maybe, they'll hop on board as well!

This recipe makes four servings and requires about 30 minutes of overall preparation time.

Here's what's inside of it:
- White wine vinegar (1) (You'll use this to sprinkle onto your food)
- Mixed greens (5 oz.)
- Chopped parsley (0.5 cup, fresh)
- Jumbo-sized shrimp with shells on them (1 lb.)
- Sea salt
- Red peppers (1 nip)
- Sliced garlic (2 cloves)
- Lemon zest (4 strips)
- Extra-virgin olive oil (0.5 cup but more may be needed for glazing

Here's how you make it:
- Place the garlic, lemon zest, oil, red pepper, and 0.24 tsp of salt into a smaller pot with a medium heat under it. It'll take about 2-3 minutes for it to sizzle.
- Preheat your large skillet with a medium heat under it. Brush a small coating of olive oil inside it. Strategically, place the shrimp in your large skillet and let it cook. Cover them up. It'll take about 3-5 minutes. Shrimp should be a light, milky color.
- Take the shrimp, once done, to your large bowl. Now, you'll add the parsley and lemon oil and toss about until all contents are well mixed.
- Divide your greens into four separate places.
- Place the shrimp strategically on top of the greens.
- Put some extra dressing in your bowl, at the bottom of it, and over the greens.

Sprinkle the white wine vinegar onto it to your liking. (We recommend one sprinkle, tasting and then increasing from there.)
- Special note: Shrimp can be replaced with a vegan/vegetarian option such as hemp-based tofu or grain-free tempeh you'll have to dice.

Chicken Soup with Shirataki Rice

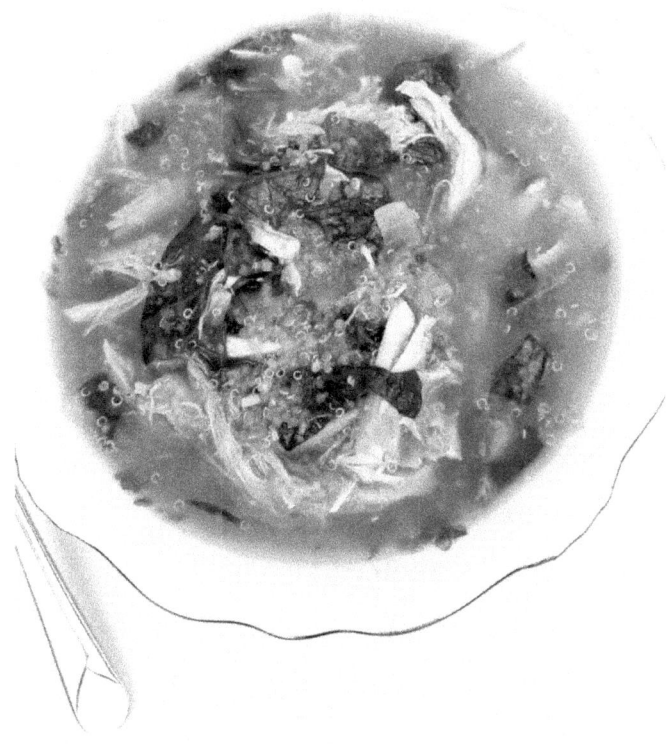

This isn't the same chicken and soup your mom gave you as a kid. In the lectin-free meal, we bring in the home comfort of a sick day with the light changing knowledge of eating healthier brings you.

This recipe will take you about 25-30 minutes to complete the preparation and cooking time. It serves about four people.

Here's what's inside of it:
- Parmigiano-Reggiano (grated for serving to your desired amount)
- Baby spinach (5 oz)
- Cooked and shredded pastured chicken (12 oz)
- Sea salt (to your desired amount)
- Black pepper (to your desired amount)
- Choice of broth (6 cups)
- Fresh rosemary (1 sprig)
- Chopped garlic (4 cloves)
- Large sliced onion (1)
- Olive oil (3 tbsp)
- Shirataki rice (1 pk)

Here's how you make it:

- Be sure to drain and rinse your shirataki rice with warm water. If you want to, boil it for 2 minutes to dry it out.
- Grab a large soup pot and heat your oil over medium-high heat.
- Add your sliced onions and cook them, constantly stirring them for about 6-8 minute. Take your garlic and rosemary, add it into the concoction, and stir it around for about 2 minutes. You should smell them incorporated into the meal.
- Get your brother and add it in with 0.5 teaspoon of salt and 0.25 teaspoon of pepper. Bring everything to a boil, lower the heat, and let your meal simmer for about 10-15 minutes.
- Add the spinach, rice, and chicken in and stir it until the chicken is warmed up and the spinach as darkened and wilted in those soup. It'll take about 3 to 5 minutes for it to do so.

- Pour the soup into four bowls and sprinkle whatever desired amount of Parmigiano on top. Enjoy!

Escarole and Shrimp Salad

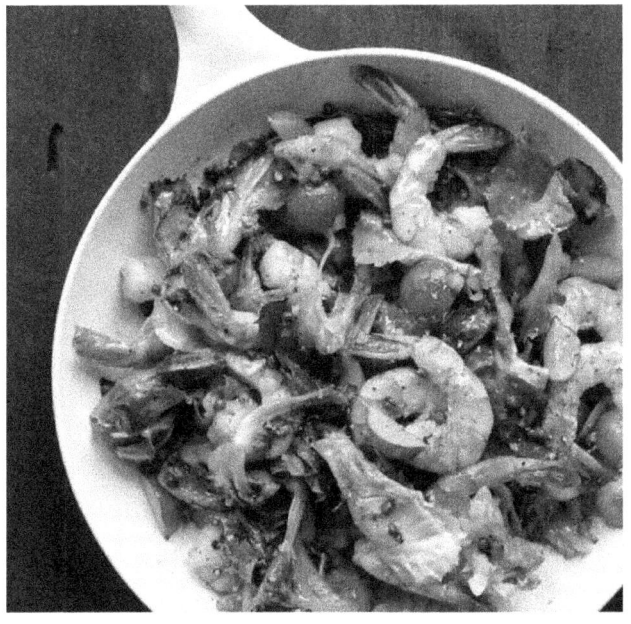

Again, with the shrimp! We can't get enough of the shrimp! This time around, we make a salad that not even the most hesitantly antisalad eater will be able to say no to.

This recipe will take you about 15 minutes to complete, including the preparation time. It makes 2-4 servings.

Here's what you'll need to toss together for the salad:
- Quartered radishes (1 bunch)
- A sliced red onion (0.50)
- The torn leaves of an escarole (1 head)
- Shrimp with the tail still on, fully cooked (1 lb.)
- Contents should all be tossed about in a larger bowl until they're mixed well with one another

To make your Caper-herb Vinaigrette, you'll need to whisk these ingredients together:

- Pepper and salt (this will vary depending on salty or savory you want your vinaigrette
- Extra-virgin olive oil (0.25 cup)
- White wine vinegar (2 tbsp)
- Dijon mustard (1 tsp)
- Chives that have been chopped (2 tbsp)
- Capers (2 tbsp)
- Shallot that's been chopped well (1)
- Mix contents into a bowl

Once both are done, pour vinaigrette over the salad and toss until contents are coated with. Mix these contents together and add salt or pepper as needed. Enjoy!

Spinach and Steak Salad

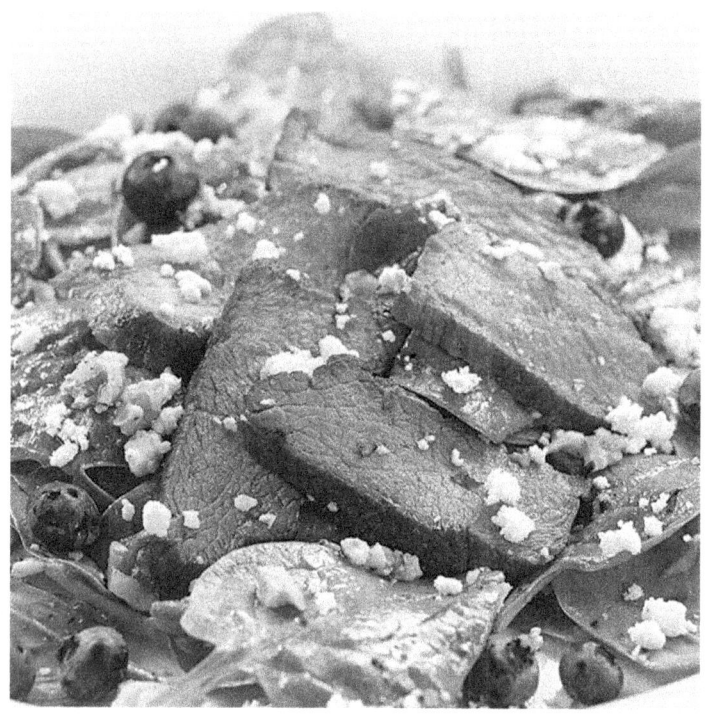

If you want to stay on the meat eater's train, then this recipe is for you! Not only do you get to continue to eat one of your favorite meats, but you get to do it knowing that you're bettering yourself.

This recipe will take you about 15 minutes to complete, including the preparation time. It makes 2-4 servings.

Here's what you'll be tossing together:
- Shirataki rice that's been drained and rinsed (1 cup)
- Roasted pine nuts (2 tbsp)
- Baby spinach (5 oz)
- The grass-fed steak that's been cooked and sliced. You can make it with medium-rare beef, but it is completely up to you. (1 lb.)

Here's what you need to make your yogurt dressing. Whisk these items together:
- Pepper and salt to your own personal preference
- Whole sheep or goat's milk yogurt (1 cup)
- Thyme leaves (2 tsp)
- Red wine vinegar (2 tbsp)

Roasted Cobb Salad

Cobb salads aren't just for the lectin-eating people of the world. Here's how to make your own version of the traditional salad.

This recipe takes a total of 20-30 minutes to complete, including the preparation and cooking time. It serves 2-4 servings.

Here's how you make the chicken and romaine: Your oven should be preheated at 450 degrees Fahrenheit. Get two boneless, skinless chicken breast halves and three large hearts of romaine (that have been halved longways) and brush them both with olive oil. When they're glazed, season them with pepper, cumin, salt, and chili powder. Start off lightly. Bake the chicken by themselves on the parchment paper in a baking sheet for about 10 minutes. Grab your romaine lettuce, cut it side down, and arrange them around your chicken. Put them together in the oven for another 5-10 minutes. Lettuce should be brown at the edges, and the chicken should be thoroughly cooked. Let them cool, and then, you'll want to chop the hearts and chicken into forkable sizes for the salad.

Serve each of the following components in heaping mounds on a serving platter:
- Crumbled goat's cheese (4 oz)
- Sliced, large and ripe avocados (2)
- Chopped scallions (1 bunch)
- Sliced, hard-boiled eggs (2)
- Chopped roasted romaine hearts (see above)
- Diced, cooked chicken (see above)

Here's how you'll make your Adobo cream dressing:
Whisk the follow ingredients together in a bowl and pour delicately over your delicious salad:
- 1/2 cup sour cream (0.50 cup)
- 1/4 cup heavy cream (0.25 cup)
- Juice from a squeezed lime (1)

- Red wine vinegar (1 tbsp)
- Adobo sauce from canned chipotles (1 tbsp)
- Salt (1 tsp)
- Cumin (1 tsp)

Meatball and Bok Choy Salad

We even have a recipe for your pork lovers out there. Bet you didn't think that you could eat meatballs again on this diet huh? Well, think again! Read below to find out more.

This recipe takes a total of 20-30 minutes to complete, including the preparation and cooking time. It serves 2-4 servings.

Here's how you'll you make the pork meatballs for your salad:
Grab one pound of ground pork and combine it with 2 cloves of chopped garlic and a generous sprinkle of salt and pepper. Mold the mixture until it makes 20 one-inch meatballs. Get 2 tablespoons of olive oil into a large skillet and heat it up over medium-high heat. Cook your meatballs, making sure to occasionally turn them. They should be brown and ready in about 8-10 minutes. Put them on a plate and leave the

pan drippings behind. Add 2 cups of sliced shiitake mushrooms into the skillet and sauté them for around 3-5 minutes.

Here's what you'll toss together for your salad:
- Your cooked meatballs
- Chopped and salted macadamia nuts (0.25 cup)
- Chopped fresh cilantro (0.50 cup)
- Thinly sliced scallions (4)
- Your sautéed shiitake mushrooms
- Heads of baby bok choy (6)

Once all the contents are in a bigger bowl, toss them about until they're mixed. Set aside.

Here's what you'll need to make your red pepper vinaigrette:

Whisk the following ingredient together in a smaller bottle:
- Red pepper (0.5 tsp)
- Sesame oil (1 tbsp)

- Golden monk fruit sweetener (2 tsp)
- Coconut aminos (1 tbsp)
- Lime juice (3 tbsp)

The Plant Patty Burger

A vegan burger has nothing on this gargantuan alternative of a burger. It'll wow traditional burger eats with its heartiness, and it'll make your stomach smile because it's lectin-free.

This recipe takes a total of 50 minutes, including the prep and cooking time. It serves four.

Here's what's inside of the patties:
- Cassava flour (2 tbsp)
- Pepper and salt
- Hungarian paprika (1 tsp)
- Fresh parsley (1 bunch)
- Fresh basil (1 bunch)
- Heaped caps chopped mushrooms (2) or 2 Big portobello mushrooms
- Big cloves of garlic (2)
- Chopped red onions (0.50 – 1 cup)
- Cubed red beetroots (2 cups)
- Walnuts (2 cups)

Here's what's inside of the sauce:
- Pepper to your personal preference
- Lemon juice (0.50 tsp)
- Bourbon (1 tsp)
- Prepared horseradish (2 tbsp)
- Heaped Kimchi Sriracha sauce (1 tbsp)
- Avocado mayonnaise (2 tbsp)

Here's what you'll need for stacking:
- Prosciutto di Parma (2 slices)
- Parmigiano Reggiano (Shavings to your personal preference)
- Red onion (A few rings)
- Pickles (A few slices)
- Portobello mushrooms (4; one for each burger as there will be no top; you'll need oil for cooking them too)
- Fresh lettuce that's been washed and dried in advanced (1 head)

Here's how you'll make it:

- Heat your oven to 350 degrees Fahrenheit.
- Make the patties by mixing all the ingredients into your food processor until it's minced. It should still have some texture to it.
- Form your patties, add them to a sheet pan, and cook them in the oven for about 20 minutes.
- Get your portobello mushrooms. Put them on a sheet pan and add some avocado oil or olive oil and salt and pepper to your liking. Cook them in the oven at the same time as your patties. They should take about 20 minutes as well.
- In the meantime, prepare your sauce by mixing all your ingredients together in a smaller bowl.
- When your mushrooms and patties are finally done, start putting together your burgers.

- Raise the oven temperature to 460 degrees Fahrenheit, place four Prosciutto di Parma slices on a sheet pan and put it into the oven. They should become a bit crisp while you make your burger. Be sure to check on them frequently.
- To put it all together, start with a slice of mushroom, then add your lettuce, your onion, burger patty, your sauce, cheese, pickles, and top with a crispy prosciutto.

Lectin-Free, Vegan Taco "Meat"

Do you want to celebrate Taco Tuesdays still? Well, this recipe will help you be able to make some tasty alternatives to the traditional taco meat. You'll love it! We promise!

This recipe takes of a total time of 5 minutes to make, including the preparation time. It makes 1.5 cups.

Here's what you'll need to make the recipe:
- Organic chili powder (1 tsp)
- Organic chipotle powder (1 tsp)
- Organic cumin powder (1 tsp)
- Himalayan pink salt (0.50 tsp)
- Organic extra-virgin olive oil (10 tsp)
- Organic walnuts (2 cups)

Here's how you'll make them:
- Combine all of your ingredients into a food processor and process it until the

walnuts are broken down into really small pieces. Be sure not to over process though.
- Adjust the seasonings to your personal preference.
- Use these for tacos, for filling in a wrap, nacho, or even for a salad!
- Store the remaining contents in a container and refrigerate.
- It'll last for a few days.
- Enjoy!

Chapter 4: Lectin-Free Dinner Recipes

Angel Hair Shirataki Noodles with Broiled Clams Over Them

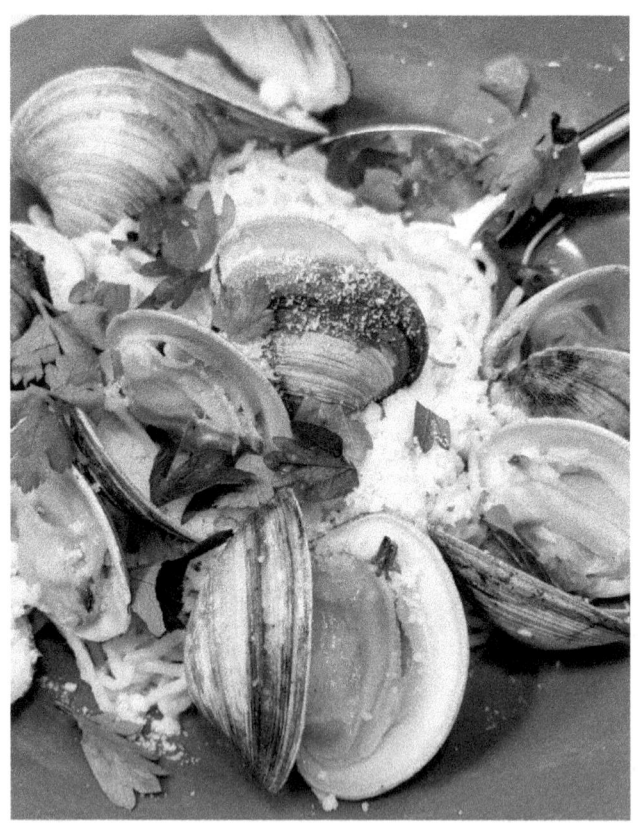

This recipe takes around 20-30 minutes to complete in both its preparation and cooking. It serves about four people.

Here's what's inside of it:
- Freshly chopped parsley (0.25 cup)
- Parmigiano-Reggiano, grated in a fine manner (0.5 cup, with more needed for when you're serving the meal)
- Italian or French-based butter (4 tbsp, in smaller cubes)
- Hard-shelled, clean-scrubbed clams (24 of them)
- Sea salt (to desired taste)
- Black pepper (to desired taste)
- Red pepper (0.25 cup)
- Crushed and peeled garlic (6 cloves)
- Seafood based broth (2 cups)
- Olive oil (1 tbsp)
- Pack of angel hair styled shirataki noodles (2 packs)

Here's how you make it:

- Drain and then rinse your shirataki noodled in warm water. Boil them for an additional 2 minutes and then dry them out if you choose to.
- Turn on your broiler's heat and make sure that the rack is roughly 6 inches from the flame. Take your oil, your butter, garlic, red pepper, and a sprinkle of salt and bring them together into a 9-by-13-inch glass baking dish. Broil the concoction until garlic is a toasty golden brown, give or take 2 minutes. Add your clams and broil it all together until the clams open up, give or take 4 to 6 minutes.
- Grab a large-sized pot, place it over medium-low heat, and put the noodle inside of it. Add your parsley, partigiano, and butter and toss the contents around until butter has melted and coated your noodles.
- Take your clams out of the oven and then put them over your noodles with butter

and garlic mix splashed on the noodles. Be sure to sprinkle any more salt, black pepper, or Parmigiano onto the meal to your liking.

Avocado and Egg Over a Noodle Bowl

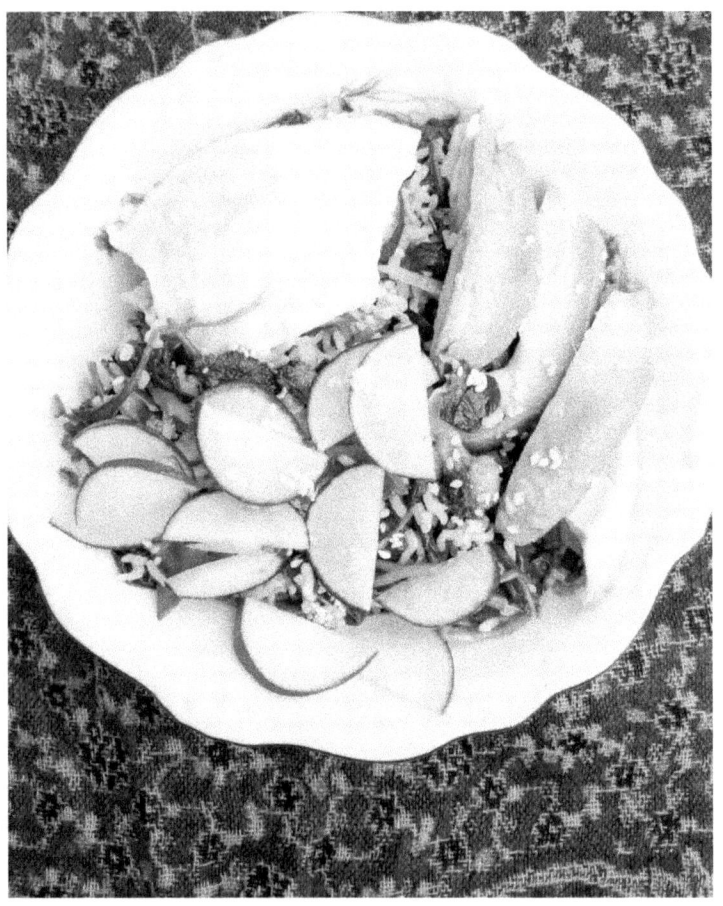

Egg noodle bowls are some of the most delicious dishes you can make, but most of the time, they contain a lot of lectins on them. Luckily, we've got a recipe here for an egg noodle bowl that'll have you smiling and continuing on the road to healthier living.

This recipe takes around 20-30 minutes to complete in both preparation and cooking. It serves about four people.

Here's what's inside it:
- Large omega-3 or fried pastured eggs (4)
- Radishes that have been thinly sliced (4)
- Avocados that have been thinly sliced (2)
- Toasted sesame seeds (2 tsp, more may be needed for dish's garnish)
- Rice vinegar (2 tbsp)
- Black pepper (0.25 tsp)
- Sea salt (0.25 tsp)
- Baby spinach (8 oz)
- Scallions that have been thinly sliced (2)
- Broccoli "crown" (1, with the pieces cut into small "trees")

- Sesame oil (0.25 cup, divided)
- Spaghetti-styled shirataki spaghetti noodles

Here's how to make it:

- Drain and then rinse your shirataki noodles in warm water. Boil them for an additional 2 minutes to dry them out if you want to.
- Place 1 tablespoon of oil into a large-sized skillet over a medium-sized heat. Cook the scallions and broccoli for about 5 minutes.
- Afterward, add your pepper, salt, and spinach and toss the contents about for a minute.
- Add your noodles and toss over the heat for around 2 minutes.
- Take your sesame seeds, vinegar, and the rest of your oil, put them into a small bowl, and whisk them together.

- Grab four bowls and put your radishes, avocado, vegetable mix, and noodles into them in equal servings.
- Add a fried egg to the top of each bowl and sprinkle in sesame seeds for garnishment.
- Drizzle with some sesame dressing and enjoy!

Goat Cheese and Chicken Enchiladas

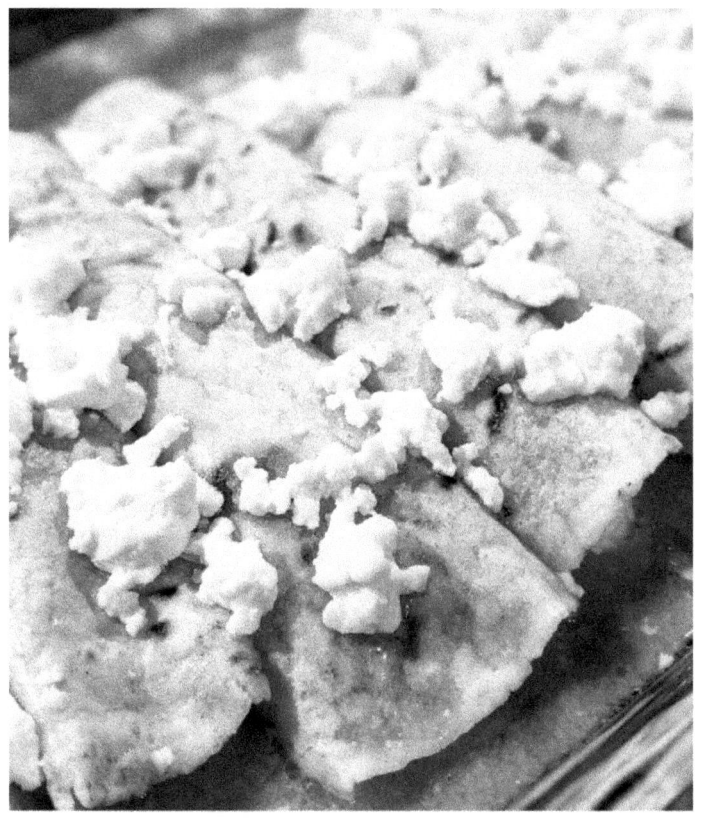

Enchiladas are one of the most celebrated food worldwide. Traditionally, it can also be one of the most carb-heavy and lectin-heavy dishes out there. As delicious as traditional enchiladas are, you're here because you want to change your life! So, here's an enchilada recipe for those nights you want to reach out for something with a southwestern flare.

This recipe takes around 45 minutes in total to make, including the preparation time. It makes eight pieces of enchilada.

Here's what's inside of it:
- A hot sauce of your choice for when you're serving it
- Freshly chopped cilantro (amount varies on individual preference)
- Cassava flour tortillas that have been warmed (8)
- Paprika (0.25 tsp)
- Dried oregano (0.5 tsp)
- Ground cumin (0.5 tsp)

- Granular sweetener (1 tsp)
- Coconut aminos (1 tsp)
- Apple cider vinegar (3 tsp)
- Peeled garlic (4 cloves)
- Crumbled goat cheese (8 oz)
- Chopped white onion (1)
- Chopped shiitake mushrooms (8 oz)
- Olive oil (2 tbsp)

Here's how you make it:

- Grab a large nonstick skillet and put it over medium-high heat. Pour your oil in and heat it up.
- Add your onions and mushrooms and let them cook. Be sure to stir them often. They should soften, which will take roughly 6-8 minutes.
- Add your 0.25 teaspoon of pepper, your 0.50 teaspoon of salt, 0.50 cup of broth, and your chicken.
- Lower the heat to medium and cook the contents.

- Stir frequently. A lot of the liquid should be absorbed. It should take roughly 3-4 minutes.
- Take the contents, pour it into a bigger bowl, and put in half of your goat cheese into it.
- You'll want to make your adobo sauce now. Grab your food blender and take your paprika, oregano, cumin, sweetener, 2 teaspoons of sea salt, coconut aminos, cider vinegar, garlic, and the remains of your broth together and pulse them. The contents should be liquidy and smooth and may take up to 3 minutes to create.
- Take 0.50 cup of your adobo sauce and pour it into the bottom of your 9-by-13 glass baking dish.
- Grab your 0.25 measuring cup and use it to scoop up your mushroom content into the tortillas. Roll each of them up and place them with seam side toward the pan to keep them from opening up.

- Once they're all rolled up, be sure to pour the remaining sauce on top of them to smother them. Sprinkle the last remains of your goat cheese on top as well.
- Bake your enchiladas at 350 degrees Fahrenheit for about 15 minutes. Check them at 5-minute intervals just to be sure! The cheese should be melted and the saucing bubbling.
- Sprinkle on your choice hot sauce and cilantro. Enjoy!

The Tuna Helper Remix!

Now, it's time to take it back to childhood. Hamburger and Tuna Helpers were all the rage back then. They were easy to make, and they were tasty to eat. But times have changed. That doesn't mean that you can't make your own version of Tuna Helper! Read below for more.

This recipe takes a total of 20-30 minutes, including the preparation and cooking time. It yields about four servings.

Here's what you'll need for the recipe:
- Capello's Fettucine or another noodle substitute (one 9-oz box)
- Canned tuna with low mercury that's been finely chopped (two 5-oz cans)

Here's what you'll need for the roasted broccoli:
- Broccoli florets (1.5-2 lbs.)

- Avocado oil (1 tbsp)
- Salt and pepper (to your personal preference)

Here's what you'll need for the sauce
- Coconut oil, or avocado oil (2 tbsp)
- Finely chopped onion (0.75 cup)
- Minced garlic (1 tbsp)
- Cassava flour (3 tbsp)
- Coconut milk can or an alternative milk, such as unsweetened almond (one 13.5-oz can)
- Chicken broth or vegetable broth (10.5 oz)
- Salt (1 tsp)
- Ground pepper (to your liking)

Here's how you make it:

How to make the roasted broccoli:
- Preheat your oven to 400 degrees Fahrenheit.

- Chop your broccoli into smaller florets and put in a bowl with your avocado oil. Lightly salt and pepper the mix.
- Transfer to it to your parchment paper-lined baking sheet. Make sure it's large enough to allow for one layer.
- Roast the contents for about 20 minutes in your preheated oven.
- Grab a pot, get your pasta water on the burner, and bring it to a boil.
- Chop your canned tuna contents or blend it in your food processor. Then set it aside.

How to make the sauce:
- Heat your butter over medium heat in a large saucepan. Add your onion. Cook them together on high, making sure you're stirring every so often for about 5 minutes until the content is soft. Add your garlic and cook it for an additional 30-60 seconds until there's a little fragrance.

- Add your cassava flour to your onion content.
- Lower the heat to medium-low.
- Continue to cook it, making sure that you're stirring frequently for about a minute. The flour should turn to a golden-brown color.
- Add your coconut milk and broth. Put the heat back up to medium-high and stir the contents until it begins bubbling. Lower the heat once again. Maintain the soft boil for 2-3 minutes until the sauce thickens.
- Turn off heat.
- Add your desired amount of salt and pepper to your tuna. Mix them all together to combine them. Cover it to keep it warm.
- Boil your choice of pasta, depending on the instructions of your pasta. Then drain them.
- Add your roasted broccoli and pasta to your sauce and toss them all together.

- Sprinkle your food with Parmigiano-Reggiano if you want and serve.

You can choose from quite a few different types of noodles: broccoli stem noodles, sweet potato noodles, or shirataki noodles. Stir-fry veggie noodles for a few minutes until bright and crisp-tender or boil shirataki noodles per the package and THEN stir-fry for a few minutes until dry.

Shepherd's Pie

Another heartwarming dish straight from your mother's kitchen, but with a change in ingredients. This way, you'll be able to get all warm and cozy but also be able to stay on track and get the body you've always wanted!

This recipe will take a total of 1 hour and 5 minutes including both the prep and cooking time. It makes about four servings.

Here what you'll need to make the recipe:
- Salt and pepper to your own personal taste
- Goat's milk (0.50 cup)
- Thyme with stems taken off (3 sprigs)
- Pastures butter (6 tbsp)
- Whole garlic with skins on (3 cloves)
- Cauliflower florets (7 oz)
- Italian parsley that's been chopped (2 tbsp)

- Whole and chopped sweet potatoes (2)
- Largely diced celery stalk (1)
- Beef broth (0.50)
- Chopped and peeled carrot (1 large)
- A while chopped yellow onion (1)
- Ground lamb (1 lb.)
- Olive oil (1 tbsp)

Here's how you make it

- Preheat the oven to 375 degrees Fahrenheit.
- Chop your sweet potatoes, carrot, and onions.
- Heat a pot (cast iron pot is recommended) with olive oil over medium-high heat.
- Put in the sweet potatoes and carrots for about 10 minutes.
- Once your oven is preheated and ready, get your cauliflower florets and put them on a baking sheet alongside the garlic. Sprinkle them with olive oil and season

them with the desired amount of salt and pepper.
- Put them in the oven and bake them for about 10-15 minutes. Cauliflower should be softened.
- In the meantime, chop the celery and Italian parsley. Add onions and celery to the pot and stir the vegetable mixture.
- Add your lamb and make sure you break up the ground meat as you stir it in. The ground meat should be broken up into small pieces.
- Continue to cook the contents until the meat is a rich brown.
- Take out your cauliflower from the oven and set aside. Let it cool. Keep your oven on.
- Add your broth and herbs (keep a few fresh thyme leaves to use as garnishes for the pies in the end).
- Reduce your heat to a simmer.

- Season with salt and pepper. This depends on how much you personally want.
- Once the cauliflower and garlic are cool, remove the garlic skins and get rid of them.
- Spoon the cauliflower and garlic to your blender.
- Add your goat milk and melted butter. Blend the contents until it is smooth.
- This should take a little less than a minute.
- Stir the meat and the vegetables together until the contents have thickened. There shouldn't be that much liquid left.
- Pour your meat mixture into the four of your ramekins.
- Top each meat-filled ramekin with the cauliflower mixture and place each ramekin on a cookie sheet and bake for 30-35 minutes.

- Once the pies have baked, let them cool for 5-10 minutes. Garnish with fresh thyme leaves and serve.

Caesar Salad (Lectin-Free Version)

Everyone's favorite salad can still be your favorite with this recipe!

This recipe takes a total time of 30 minutes to create and contains about two servings.

Here's what's in it:

What you'll need for the Caesar salad:
- One or two sprinkles of salt
- Liquid Stevia (6 drops)
- Dijon mustard (1 tsp)
- Nutrient-rich yeast (2 tbsp)
- Lemon juice (2 tbsp)
- Extra virgin olive oil (5-6 tbsp)
- Minced smaller garlic (2 cloves)
- Pressure-cooked garbanzo beans (0.75 cup)
- Romaine lettuce (1 large head)

What you'll need for the Italian crusted tempeh:
- Black pepper (0.13 tsp)
- Italian seasoning (0.25 tsp)
- Truffle salt or sea salt (0.25 tsp)
- Nutrient-rich yeast (2 tsp)
- Olive oil (2 tbsp)
- Tempeh (6 oz)

Here's how to make it:
- Here is how to make the dressing: Combine your chickpeas, garlic, 5 tablespoons of olive oil, lemon, yeast, mustard, stevia, and salt into your food processor or your personal-sized blender and blend the contents until it is smooth. Make sure to add another tablespoon of olive oil if your dressing is too thick to blend correctly.
- Take your dressing, put it into a container, and place it in your fridge for about 30 minutes, but the time can extend to an hour depending on the fridge's temperature.

Here's how you prepare the lettuce:
- Cut the head of romaine into large yet bite-sized pieces. Do this by cutting the head down the center vertically, then rotate at a 90° angle, and make another vertical cut down the center. Finally, cut the head horizontally across the head into sections about 1-inch thick until you reach the bottom of the head.
- Grab it and put it in a large raised colander and rinse it thoroughly with some cold water, rubbing off any noticeable grime. Place your colander into a larger bowl and put the entire thing in the fridge while prepping your tempeh.

Here's how you prepare the tempeh:
- Grab a small bowl and mix together yeast, truffle salt, pepper, and Italian seasonings. Set it aside for now.

- Add one block of tempeh and enough water to rise 0.75 of the way up with the tempeh in a medium no-stick pan over high heat. Bring it to a boil. Stir it until all the water has evaporated. Then transfer your tempeh to a cutting board and lower the heat to medium.
- Evenly sprinkle your spice mixture onto each side of tempeh and pat down with a gentle hand to ensure it's sticky.
- Pour 2 tablespoons of olive oil into your pan. Once the oil shimmers, put your tempeh and cook them on each side until they have a golden-brown look to them. It'll be roughly 2-3 minutes per side. Turn off the heat, transfer contents to a cutting board, and cut them into strips of your personally desired thickness. Set it aside for now.

Here's how to put the salad together:
- Grab a large mixing bowl and put a majority of the lettuce together alongside

all of the dressing for about 1 minute. The dressing should be evenly laid upon the leaves. If there is enough dressing left, then add the rest of the leaves and mix it together.

- Dispense your dressed lettuce among two plates and serve with each place with equal amounts of tempeh strips. The dressing will last in the fridge for about five days. Salad my wilt if you save it, so you should eat it while it's still fresh.

Shrimp and Broccoletti Stir-Fry Over Toasted Sesame Cauliflower Rice

We promise that you won't be missing your traditional rice once you've gotten a hold of this cauliflower "rice." Just wait till you add the stir-fry and really make it exciting!

The total time it'll take to prepare and cook this recipe is 30 minutes. It contains four servings.

Here's what you'll need to make this recipe:
- Unsalted vegetable broth (0.25 cup)
- Rice vinegar (0.25 cup)
- A bag of broccoletti cut into two-inch pieces (10 oz)
- Grated fresh ginger, 2-inch piece (1 tsp)
- Minced garlic (1 tsp)
- Sliced scallions (1 bunch)
- Wild-caught shrimp that's been peeled and deveined (1 lb. raw)

- Avocado oil (3 tbsp)
- Riced cauliflower (0.50 head)

Here's how you make it:

- In a microwave-safe dish, cook your cauliflower rice for about 35 minutes. Be sure to put in the sesame seeds too.
- In the meantime, heat 1 tablespoon of your oil into a large skillet. Crank up the heat to medium-high heat.
- Add your shrimp into the pan and cook. Make sure to stir it often. It should take about 2-4 minutes to complete. Once done, put on a plate and reserve the skillet.
- Get your remaining 2 tablespoons of oil and put it into the reserved skillet.
- Add your broccoletti, ginger, and scallions. Stir and cook the contents until your broccoletti is tender. This should take 8-10 minutes.

- Get your vinegar and vegetable broth and stir them in. Be sure to toss it frequently and make sure that your vegetables are covered in the sauce. This will take about 2 minutes.
- Finally, add your shrimp and toss the contents for an additional 1 minute.
- Put the cauliflower rice in a bowl first and then serve your stir-fry over it. Sprinkle on some additional sesame seeds, to your liking.
- Enjoy!

Apricot Balsamic Chicken

This recipe is perfect for those nights when you want to do something a little different, or you want to impress someone! What's most impressive is that it's lectin-free!

This recipe has a total preparation and cooking time of 35 minutes. It serves four servings.

Here's what you'll need for this recipe:
- Butter lettuce (1 head, torn into pieces)
- Fresh lemon juice (1 tsp)
- One-inch Parmigiano-Reggiano cubes (2)
- Walnuts or pine nuts (0.25 cup)
- Basil leaves, fresh and pack (1 cup)
- Extra-virgin olive oil (0.50 cup)
- Pastured chicken cutlets (8)
- Avocado oil
- Himalayan sea salt
- Ground ginger (0.50 tsp)
- Balsamic vinegar (0.25 cup)

- Apricot preserves, no sugar added (0.25 cup)

Here's how you'll make it:
- Heat your grill to medium-low heat.
- Grab a large bowl and combine your preserves, vinegar, ginger, and 0.75 teaspoon of sea salt. Set aside 0.25 cup of the mixture.
- Add your cutlets to the bowl and toss the contents around until you coat them. Let them sit for about 10 minutes.
- In the meantime, grab your blender and pulse together the olive oil, basil, pine nuts, cheese, and lemon juice until they are all blended well.
- Grill your cutlets until they're cooked all the way through. This will take about 13-15 minutes. Make sure to turn them occasionally and baste them with your reserved mixture within the last ¾ minutes of them grilling.

- Divide your lettuce among the plates and sprinkle with the basil-pesto vinaigrette.
- Serve it with the chicken cutlets and enjoy!

Chicken Mushroom Limes

If you're looking for something a little zesty and a little creamy, then give this recipe a shot!

This recipe has a total preparation and cooking time of 45 minutes. It contains about four servings.

Here's what you'll need for the recipe:
- Lime wedges (for serving)
- Olive oil (for the grill)
- Black pepper
- Himalayan sea salt
- Ground cumin (0.50 tsp)
- Extra-virgin olive oil (2 tbsp)
- Limes (2 of them cut into 8 pieces each)
- Small, red onion (1, cut into 1.5-inch pieces)
- Portobello mushrooms (2, cut into 1.5-inch pieces)

- Pastured, boneless, skinless chicken thighs (0.75 lb.)
- Riced cauliflower (1 head)

Here's how you'll make it:
- Preheat your grill and grill pan to medium heat.
- Cook your cauliflower rice in the microwave in a covered dish for about 5 minutes.
- Let it sit for another 5 minutes and then fluff it with a fork. Add the lime zest.
- In the meantime, grab a large bowl and toss 0.25 teaspoon of black pepper, 0.75 teaspoon of salt, cumin, with oil, limes, onion, mushrooms, and chicken.
- Lightly oil the grill pan on the grill via a paper towel.
- Grill the chicken and vegetable concoction making sure to stir it occasionally. Chicken should be cooked through, and

the onions should be tender. It'll take about 15-18 minutes.
- Serve it with your "rice" and lime wedges and enjoy!

Sirloin Steak Leeks

Easily one of our favorite lectin-free steak recipes, this one is guaranteed to at least pique the interest of your meat-loving, lectin-free diet skeptic friend or family member.

This recipe has a total preparation and cooking time of 20 minutes. It serves four servings.

Here's what you need to make this recipe:
- Himalayan sea salt (1 tsp)
- Water (tbsp)
- Red wine vinegar (2 tbsp)
- Garlic coarsely chopped (1 clove)
- Dried oregano (2 tsp)
- Baby arugula (2 cups, loosely packed)
- Baby greens (5 cups)
- Trimmed leeks (1 bunch)
- Extra-virgin olive oil (6 tbsp, divided)
- Black pepper (0.75 teaspoon)

- Sirloin grass-fed steak (1 lb., cut into 2 pieces)

Here's how you'll make it:
- Heat up your grill to medium.
- Season your steak with pepper and coat it with 1 teaspoon of oil. Grill it, turning it once, until a thermometer inserted in the center of each one registers 130 degrees Fahrenheit. It'll take roughly 5-7 minutes on each side for a medium rare steak. It's longer if you want it well done.
- Remove them, let them rest for about 5 minutes, and then slice them against the grain.
- In the meantime, toss your leak in a 1 tablespoon of oil. Grill them over an indirect heat, around your steak, making sure to turn them occasionally. In 6-7 minutes, they should be charred and tender.
- Remove them and roughly chop them up.

- Pulse your arugula, salt, water, vinegar, last of your oil, garlic, and oregano together in a blender until it's smooth.
- Divide your steaks, greens, and leeks onto four plates. Drizzle them with the dressing and enjoy!

Dijon Salmon Cakes

Perfect for those summer days when you're craving some salmon and want a savory twist to it. Fair warning: you may want to eat this recipe up on our own!

The total time this recipe takes to prepare, and cook is 45 minutes. It makes around four servings.

Here's what's inside the recipe:
- Dijon mustard (2 tbsp and more for serving)
- Roughly chopped scallions (2)
- Alaskan sockeye salmon (1, skinned)
- Sea salt and black pepper
- Extra-virgin olive oil (2 tbsp, divided)
- Fresh mint that's been torn (0.25 cup)
- Kalamata olives (0.50 cup)
- Organic vegetable broth (2 cups)
- Millet (1 cup)

Here's how you make it:

- Combine your millet and broth into a medium-sized saucepan. Put the heat up to medium-high and bring contents to a boil.
- Turn the heat to low and simmer with it covered for about minutes. Add the olives, mint, 1 tablespoon of olive oil, and 0.50 teaspoon of salt and pepper each.
- Get your salmon and wrap it in a paper towel, making sure to squeeze out any excess water. Pulse the salmon, 0.25 teaspoon of pepper, 0.40 teaspoon of salt, and scallions together in a food processor or blender until all of it is chopped up finely.
- Take the salmon and put it in a bowl and mix in 0.50 cup of cooked millet and your Dijon mustard. Make 8 different patties.
- Heat 1 tablespoon of oil into a large skillet over medium heat.

- Cook the patties until opaque. It'll be about 2 minutes on each side.
- Serve them warm with the remains of the millet and some steamed greens. You can also store them in your fridge for snacks or for a lunch. They hold for about three days.

Chapter 5: Lectin-Free Dessert Recipes

Who says you can't have something sweet while you're on the lectin-free diet? With these lectin-free dessert recipes, satisfying that sweet tooth couldn't be any simpler!

Summer-Time Strawberry Short Cake

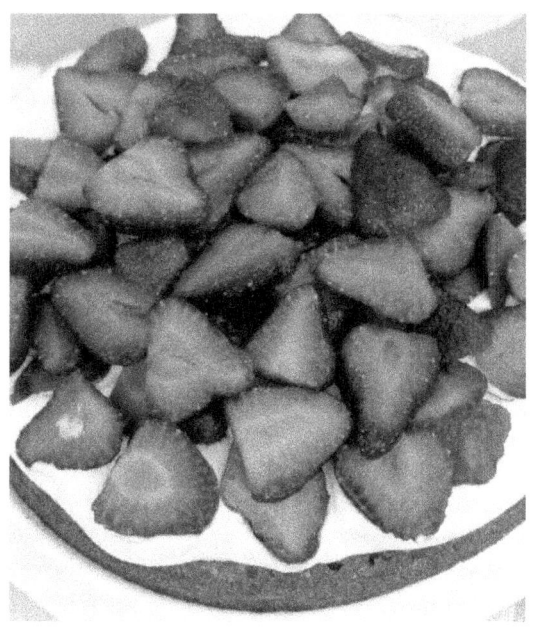

This recipe takes a total preparation and cooking time of one hour and contains about 8 servings.

Here's what's inside the cake's topping:
- Fresh strawberries that have been sliced and prepped (1 qt)
- Vanilla extract (0.5 tsp)
- Your choice of yacon syrup or raw honey (1 tbsp)
- Your choice of organic or grass-fed heavy cream product

Here's what's inside the actual cake:
- Baking soda (0.75 tsp)
- Sea salt (0.50 tsp)
- Arrowroot starch (3 tbsp)
- Tigernut flour (0.3 cup)
- Coconut flour (0.3 cup)
- Vanilla extract (0.5 tsp)
- Zest of a lemon grated (0.5 of the lemon)
- Stirred up coconut cream (0.5 cup)

- Your choice of large omega-3 based eggs or large pastured eggs (3 at room temperature)
- Golden monk fruit sweetener (0.25 cup)
- Your choice of Italian butter or unsalted French butter (8 tbsp at room temperature)

Here's how you make it:
- First, preheat your oven to 350 degrees Fahrenheit.
- Butter the bottom part of a rounded, 8-inch cake pan. Then line up the pan with parchment paper. Be sure to wipe it with yet another layer of butter and sprinkle it with a small thin layer of flour.
- Beat your sweetener and butter in your mixer on a higher speed. Contents should come out fluffy and light. Decrease the speed to medium and then add your eggs one by one.

- Add your vanilla, lemon zest, and coconut cream into the mix until the concoction if blended well. Stop your machine and scrap the sides of the bowl if contents on the sides are not mixing with the other contents.
- Sift the contents of your baking soda, sea salt, arrowroot starch, tigernut flour, and coconut flour together.
- Combine your butter mixture with your sifted content and let them mix together on a lower speed. Contents should look smooth when done.
- Carefully pour your batter into your pan and smooth out the top of it with your spatula. Be sure to hit your pan against the counter a couple of times to make the battle settle.
- Cook your batter for roughly 35 minutes or until your toothpick comes out of it clean.

- Let the cake cool in the pan for around 30 minutes.
- When cooled off, flip the cake onto a cooling rack and let the cake finish cooling until it's room temperature.
- Bring the contents of vanilla, yacon, or honey, and your choice of cream together on high speed until you see little peaks form on top.
- Move your cake onto a platter or something else flat and place the whipped contents on top of it. Strategically place your strawberries on top in decorative patterns!

Lectin-Free Blueberry Fools

This recipe takes a total of 1 hour to create including preparation time. It contains four servings.

Here's what you'll need to make it:
- Real vanilla extract (0.5 tsp)
- Organic, heavy whipping cream (1.3 cups)
- Lemon zest and juice (0.5 lemon)
- A sprinkle of salt
- Xylitol (3 tbsp, divided)
- Blueberries (2 cups, and more for garnish later)

Here's how you make it:
- Heat up 1.5 cups of blueberries, 2 tbsp of xylitol, and a sprinkle of salt in a saucepan over medium heat.
- Bring contents to a bubble.
- Reduce heat to medium-low and cook, making sure to occasionally stir until your

blueberries soften. It should take no more than 5 minutes.
- Remove them from heat and stir in your lemon zest, juice, and the remaining 0.50 cup of blueberries, and let them cool down until they're room temperature.
- In the meantime, beat your heavy cream, the remaining tablespoon of xylitol, and vanilla together in a mixer until soft peaks begin to form.
- Put the cooled blueberry sauce into the whipped cream gently.
- Divide the contents into bowls and top them with more blueberries.
- Enjoy!

Chapter 6: Lectin-Free Snack Recipes

There's going to be those moments at night in which you're going to want to give up and just eat something—anything that's in your fridge. You're not quite hungry for a full meal, but you're still hungry. Luckily, there is where these snack recipes come in handy! They'll come to your rescue as you raid the fridge at midnight.

Coconut Wrapped Raviolis

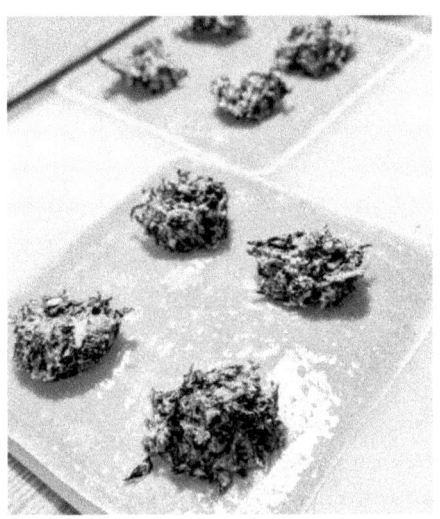

This recipe has a total of 35 minutes to prepare and complete. It takes ten larger sized raviolis.

Here's what you'll need to make the raviolis:
- Omega-3 or pastured eggs (2, they should be mixed with 1 tsp of water)
- Square shaped coconut wraps (5)
- Parmigiano-Reggiano that's been grated (0.25 cup)
- Italian mascarpone (0.25 cup)
- Spinach that's been thawed, squeezed dry and thawed (one 10-oz package)
- Extra-virgin olive oil (4 tbsp, divided)

Here's what you'll need to make the pesto:
- Extra-virgin olive oil (0.5 cup)
- Garlic (2 cloves)
- Parmigiano-Reggiano (1 oz, crumbled)
- Pine nuts (0.25 cup)
- Fresh basil (2 cups, packed)

Here's what you'll need for serving:

- Your personal choice for an additional amount of balsamic vinegar and olive oil
- Mixed salad greens (5 oz)

Here's how you make them:
- Grab a large saucepan and heat up 2 tablespoons of olive oil
- Add your spinach. Cook in the oil for about 2 minutes.
- Put contents in a bowl and then stir in the Parmigiano and the mascarpone.
- Get your cutting board and line up 2.5 wraps.
- Brush them with your water and egg mixture.
- Get a tablespoon, grab some of the fillings, and place little balls of it into the four corners of each of the wraps. For the half wrap, there should only be two. Be sure to leave a space between the balls of the mixture so that they don't stick together.

- Get your egg wash and brush the top of the other wraps. Gently place them on top of the other wraps and press around mixture, sealing the sides.
- Grab a fluted ravioli cutter and cut out four squares from the sealing and filling.
- You can also use a pizza cutter. You can either cut a square and rounded raviolis. Just makes sure ravioli stay sealed.
- Now, it's time to make your basil pesto! Simply, grab all your ingredients for the pesto and blend them together in your blender. Blend until contents are smooth.
- Get your remaining 2 tablespoons of olive oil into your pan and put it over medium heat. Fry a few raviolis at a time in the 2-3-minute interval. Be sure to flip them halfway.
- Serve them with the salad greens and pesto.
- Sprinkle on any additional balsamic vinegar or olive oil as you see fit.

Fresh Rainbow Fries (From the Oven)

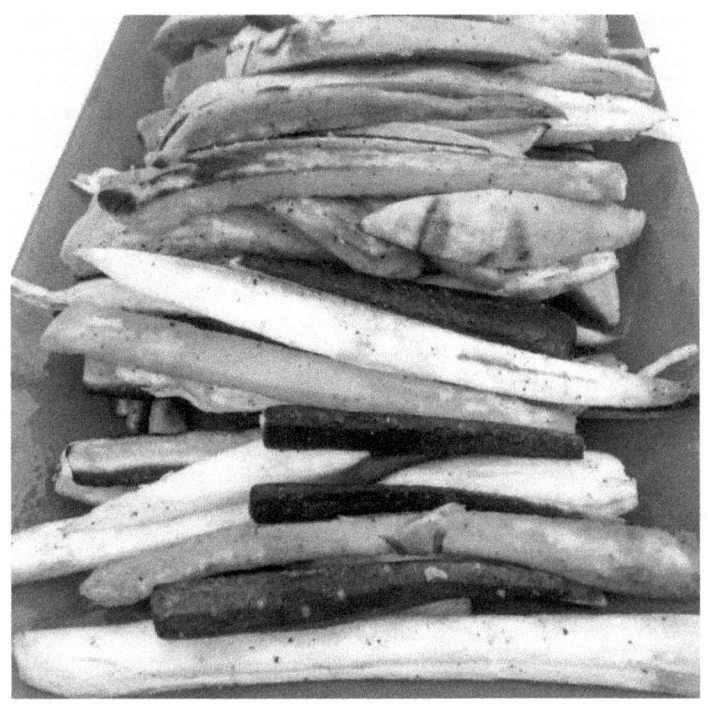

This recipe has a total time of 40 minutes for both preparations and cooking. It serves 8 people.

Here's what inside the recipe:

- Grainy mustard (3 tbsp)
- Full fat sour cream (0.75 cup)
- Black pepper
- Sea salt (2 tsp)
- Extra-virgin olive oil (3 tbsp)
- Medium-sized sweet potatoes that are cut and peeled into 0.25-inch strips (2)
- Medium-sized Yuca roots that are cut and peeled into 0.25-inch strips (2)
- Purple carrots which are quartered, halved, and peeled at a longer length (4)

Here's how you make it:

- Grab two baking sheets and place them in the top and bottom parts of the oven.
- Preheat your oven to 450 degrees Fahrenheit.
- Toss your sweet potatoes, yuca, and carrots in a bowl with your granulated garlic, salt, and a sprinkle or two of pepper (to your liking) and olive oil. Make sure to coat them well.

- Place the different sticks on baking sheets inside the oven.
- Bake the sticks until they're golden and crispy, making sure to flip them around and to put the ones on the top rack on the bottom and vice versa. Do this halfway into the overall 20 minutes.
- In the meantime, take your mustard, your cream, and a decent amount of pepper (again to your personal liking), and mix the contents into a small bowl.
- Once the fries are ready, put them on a serving plate with your dip and enjoy!

Great Mashed Potatoes Alternatives!

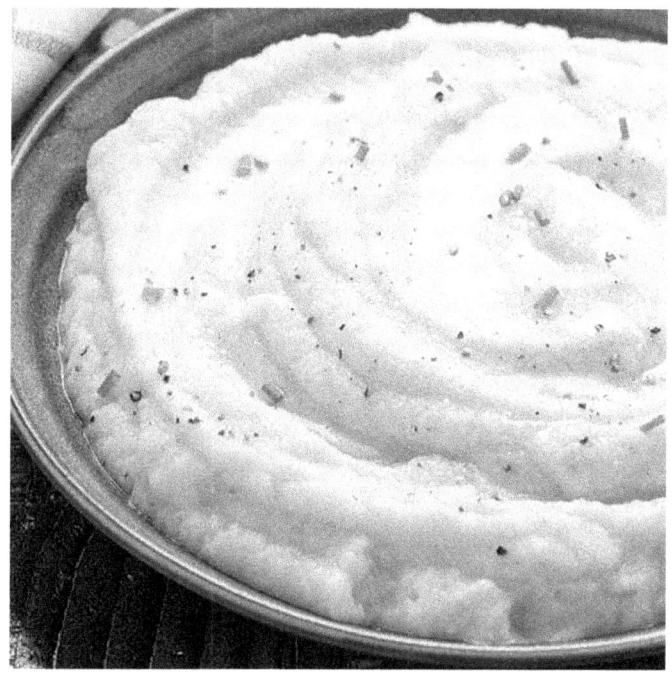

Here's how you'll make mashed cauliflower:
- Begin with 2 pounds of cauliflower florets that come from 2 large heads previously. Steam them to make the contents soft.

- Mash the cauliflower florets with 2 tablespoons of Italian or French butter. You will not need any liquid.
- Mix contents with 1.5 cups shredded Parmigiano-Reggiano cheese.
- Top your mashed "potatoes" with chopped rosemary and chives.

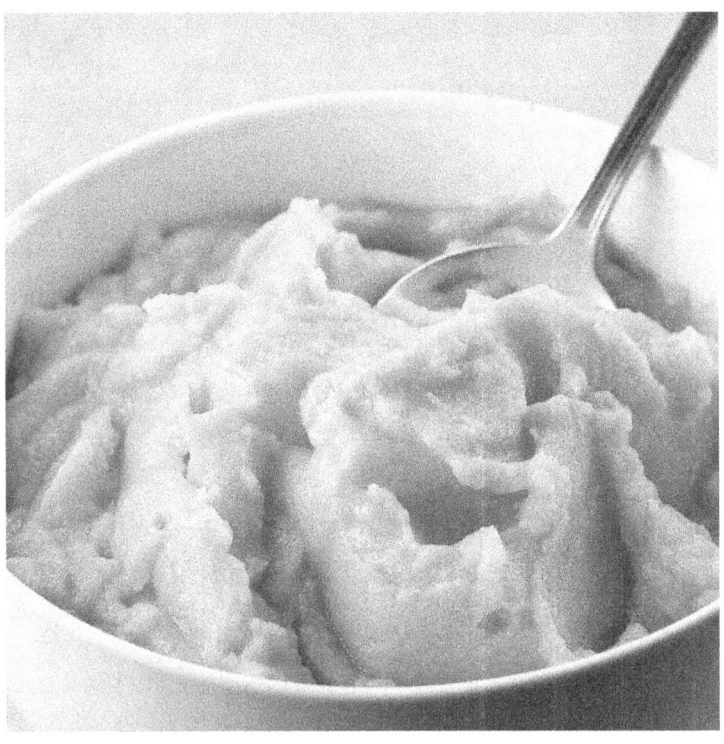

Here's how you'll make mashed (sweet) potatoes

- You'll start with your 2 pounds of sweet potatoes. Make sure they're steamed, diced, and peeled.
- Mash your soften sweet potatoes with 0.25 cup of almond milk and 4 tablespoons of a French- or Italian-styled butter.
- Mix your mashed "potatoes" into 1 teaspoon of salt, 0.50 teaspoon of cinnamon, and one sprinkle of allspice.
- Top your mashed "potatoes" with your scallions chopped pecans! Enjoy!

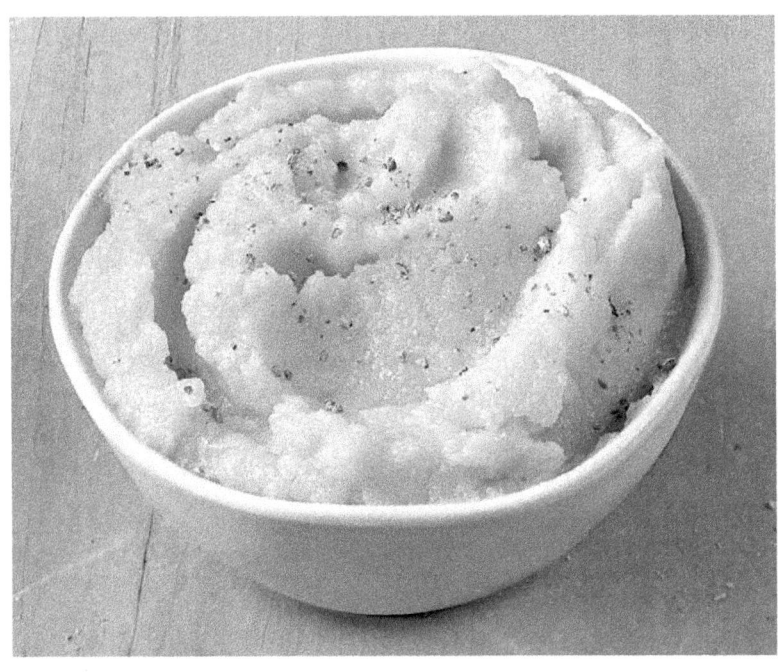

Here's how you'll make mashed parsnips

- You'll start your mashed "potatoes" with 2 pounds of parsnips. Make sure that they're peeled, diced, and steamed.
- Mash the contents with 0.25 cup of full-fat coconut milk and 4 tablespoons of French- or Italian-styled butter.
- Mix the contents with 2 cloves of minced garlic, 0.5 teaspoon of ground coriander,

0.5 teaspoon of salt, and 0.25 teaspoon of black pepper.
- Top your delicious mashed "potatoes" with your choice of chopped and fresh herbs. We recommend rosemary, sage, thyme, or mint!

Pickled Celery from the Fridge

This recipe will take over 48 hours to prepare and complete. It makes 3-5 servings.

Here's what you'll need for this recipe:
- Celery that's been rinsed with the ends chopped off and removed. Slice them long-wise into spears (5 stalks; 1 will make about 2-3 spears)
- To make the brine, get 0.75 cup of white vinegar, 3 teaspoons of sea salt, and 1.5 tablespoon of sweetener. You can also use raw honey for this.
- To make the seasoning, get one clove of garlic that's been peeled and smashed, 0.50 teaspoon of whole mustard seeds, and 0.25 black peppercorns.

Here's how you'll make this recipe:

- Grab a 16-oz glass jar or something similar to put your pickled celery in.
- Put your celery spears into the empty jar.
- Cut any of the spears so that they are not taller than the top of the jar.
- Mix together all your brine ingredients in a small bowl. Make sure to stir for about 5 minutes until your salt and sweetener dissolve. There may be some grainy particles left, but that's fine!
- Pour your brine into your jar and over the celery spears.
- Your celery should be virtually covered with the brine.
- Add your garlic clove, mustard seeds, and peppercorns into your brine and celery jar.
- Cover the contents tightly with a lid.
- Let the jar sit on the counter for 4-6 hours.

- Afterward, transfer into the refrigerator.
- Pickles will continue to brine in the fridge.
- Let stand in the fridge for about 48 hours.
- Enjoy! They will stay for roughly a week.

Multi-Seed Grain-Free Bread

This recipe has a complete time of 20-30 minutes to complete including preparation. It makes one loaf.

Here's what's in the recipe:

- Sunflower seeds (0.50 cup with more needed for topping)
- Pumpkin seeds (0.50 cup with more needed for topping)
- Sesame seeds (0.50 cup)
- Chia seeds (0.25 cup)
- Salt and pepper (0.25 tsp of each)
- Nutrient-rich yeast (1 tbsp)
- Garlic powder (1 tsp)
- Apple cider vinegar (1 tsp)
- Avocado oil (0.5 cup)
- Coconut flour (0.25 cup)
- Almond flour (1 cup)

Here's how you'll make it:

- Preheat your oven to 350 degrees Fahrenheit.
- Crack your eggs and put them in a blender with your oil and your vinegar. Blend the contents on low until they're all combined.
- Place your chia seeds and sesame seeds into a food processor or a coffee grinder and grind it until the seeds are broken down and look like coarse flour.
- Add your chia and sesame seed mixture, garlic powder, and nutritional yeast into a blender. Blend this concoction on low until they're all combined.
- Pour the contents into a large mixing bowl and slowly fold in your almond flour.
- Once almond flour is fully mixed in, start to slowly fold in coconut flour. You may not need the full 0.25 cup of coconut flour. If at any point the dough seems too thick and dry, slowly add more oil. If it

seems too wet, slowly add more coconut flour.
- Now, it's time to put your pumpkin and sunflower seeds in the food processor and roughly chop them. Mix your seeds into the dough.
- Line a loaf pan with parchment paper and add dough to the pan. If you want, top with additional seeds.
- Bake for 45 minutes and remove from the oven to cool.
- Do not slice the bread until it's fully cooled.
- Store the bread in a container in the fridge for 5 days. Put it in the freezer if you want to make it last longer. Be sure to slice it if you do go the freezer route.
- You can make a sweet bread by replacing the garlic powder and nutrient-rich yeast with nutmeg or cinnamon.

Conclusion

Thanks for making it through to the end of *LECTIN-FREE COOKBOOK: 30 Simple, Quick, and Easy Recipes to Help You Improve Your Health, Reduce Inflammation, Prevent Risk of a Disease, and Shield Your Gut from Lectin Damage*, let's hope it was informative and able to provide you with all of the tools you need to achieve your goals whatever they may be.

The next step is to grab a pan and begin the life-changing process of lectin-free dieting today!

Finally, if you found this book useful in any way, a review on Amazon is always appreciated!

Description

With the diet revolution projected by Dr. Stephen Gundry's bestseller "Plant Paradox," the lectin-free diet has taken off and proven to be to go for many people for various reasons. It's helped people change their bodies and live life without having to eat bland things.

LECTIN-FREE COOKBOOK: 30 Simple, Quick, and Easy Recipes to Help You Improve Your Health, Reduce Inflammation, Prevent Risk of a Disease, and Shield Your Gut from Lectin Damage collects 30 of the most exciting recipes around to prove that eating Lectin-free doesn't have to be taste bud death sentence!

With these recipes in your arsenal, you're going to no problem establishing and staying on the road to recovery with these lectin-free foods. Say goodbye to uncomfortable inflammation and problematic autoimmune symptoms. You'll take charge of your life and restore the years of damage.

In this book, you'll find 30 recipes that very different and very delicious. Rather it's breakfast, lunch, dinner, and snacks and desserts, we've got you covered. The cooking and preparation time keep people like you in mind—people with busy lives. So rather you're making dinner for your family or wanting to reach for a midnight snack, you'll find something you'll enjoy.

It's time to join many other people who have adopted the lectin-free diet and learn how to shield your gut from lectin damage. We'll break down the lectin diet for you as well, so you'll know all about this new diet that's turning into more than the next fad. Get your copy NOW!

www.ingramcontent.com/pod-product-compliance
Lightning Source LLC
Chambersburg PA
CBHW071712020426
42333CB00017B/2243